M. Eibl · W.R. Mayr · G.J. Thorbecke (Eds.)

**Epitope Recognition Since
Landsteiner's Discovery**

Springer

Berlin
Heidelberg
New York
Barcelona
Hong Kong
London
Milan
Paris
Tokyo

M. Eibl W.R. Mayr
G.J. Thorbecke (Eds.)

Epitope Recognition Since Landsteiner's Discovery

100 Years Since the Discovery
of Human Blood Groups

With 34 Figures and 11 Tables

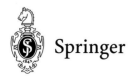 Springer

Prof. Dr. MARTHA EIBL
Immunologische Tagesklinik
Schwarzspanierstr. 15
1090 Vienna, Austria

Prof. Dr. W. R. MAYR
Allgemeines Krankenhaus der Stadt Wien
Klinische Abteilung für Blutgruppenserologie
Währinger Gürtel 18–20
1090 Vienna, Austria

G. J. THORBECKE †, MD, Ph.D.
New York University School of Medicine
Department of Pathology
550 First Avenue
New York, NY 100116, USA

ISBN 3-540-42651-5 Springer-Verlag Berlin Heidelberg NewYork

Library of Congress-Cataloging-in-Publication-Data
Epitope recognition since Landsteiner's discovery: 100 years since the discovery of human blood groups; with 11 tables / M. Eibl ... (ed.). – Berlin; Heidelberg; New York; Barcelona; Hong Kong; London; Milan; Paris; Tokyo: Springer, 2001
    ISBN 3-540-42651-5

Springer-Verlag a member of BertelsmannSpringer
Science + Business Media GmbH

http://www.springer.de

© Springer-Verlag Berlin Heidelberg 2002
Printed in Germany

Production: PRO EDIT GmbH, 69126 Heidelberg, Germany
Cover Design: design & production, 69121 Heidelberg, Germany
Printed on acid-free paper – SPIN: 10794164   27/3130Re – 5 4 3 2 1 0

In Memoriam G. Jeanette Thorbecke

† 16 November 2001

Jeanette Thorbecke, one of the organisers of the Karl-Landsteiner-Symposium on 16 July 2000, Vienna, and co-editor of these Proceedings died unexpectedly in a tragic accident.

At a time when many scientists are globally mobile and frequently change their affiliations, Jeanette Thorbecke was working at the same department and virtually in the same laboratories for over four decades. Due to the tremendous flexibility of her mind and her international outlook she was always part of and present in ongoing events of the scientific community.

Jeanette Thorbecke took pride in being an off-spring of a well-known, liberal Dutch family. She was born and educated in Holland, where she received her MD and PhD at the University of Groningen. She joined the Department of Pathology of the New York University Medical School in 1957 as a post-doctoral fellow and, after having been an instructor, assistant professor and associate professor, she became full professor in 1970 and held this position for the rest of her life.

She received a number of prestigious awards, the last of which, the Bonazinga Award, was given to her by the Society for Leukocyte Biology only a few days before her untimely death. Her official functions in different committees and societies bore testimony to the high esteem she was held in. The highlight certainly was her presidency of the American Association of Immunologists in 1990. In her presidential address she made a passionate plea to the scientific community to keep the delicate balance in funding focussed projects on the one hand without eliminating more broadly based, unconventional proposals. "What we definitely should not do is encourage the government to cut our funds by becoming more and more critical of proposals that don't fit the mold of "a sure thing", focussed project, popular subject or popular animal species."

If one tried to characterize the scientist Jeanette Thorbecke with a few words, the first quality that comes to mind was her great enthusiasm for science ever since her first encounter until her most recent projects. Her honest and critical approach was a characteristic feature of her work; she was always full of plans and ideas, for which her papers still in press or unfinished are convincing proofs.

Very early on in her scientific career, she became interested in B-cell biology and especially the architecture and the function of germinal centres. She and her co-workers made essential contributions to the field of germinal centre development in physiological and pathological conditions. One facet of her research concentrated on the aged, another on the pathogenesis of B-cell lymphomas and on regulation of T and B-cell cooperation and its role in autoimmune disease eg experimental autoimmune encephalomyelitis.

Throughout her career her research was centred on problems of basic science while at the same time never losing sight of possible medical applications and clinical significance.

She always felt great responsibility for her students and took great care that their work should be accurate and important. As she was a member of a number of study sections and committees, she was very well aware of new methodologies and evolving trends. Her students' careers were always a major concern for her but she guided them to exploit their talents rather than impose her own ideas on them. It was little surprise then that she continued cooperating with several of her former students for decades.

She was a wonderful and reliable friend. Friendship with her included challenging scientific discussions, where she always took sides when it came to innovative developments. She argued with great personal conviction but always with great respect for the ideas of others. Her objective was to provide constructive support and she only got angry if somebody failed to differentiate between significant and irrelevant questions.

Among her most striking features were the complete absence of any prejudice both in personal and in scientific matters. She totally detested any kind of injustice, was always willing to fight for her cause and steer clear of politics. She was proud of her liberal way of thinking, which was part of her family tradition.

No matter how busy she was with family and science, she always made time for the arts. Whenever time permitted, she attended classes for drawing and painting but even when time was tight, she kept contact with the arts by visiting museums and listening to lectures.

Jeanette Thorbecke was married to Dr Gerald Hochwald and had three sons.

Her love and responsibility for her family were always central to her heart. She was a loving and caring partner to her husband and was keen to and managed to transfer her intellectual craving, professional interest and responsibility to her children. And her relations with them was always led by love, affection and infinite understanding.

We will miss her and remember her as an outstanding scientist and a treasured friend.

MARTHA M. EIBL

Opening Address

Dr. Thorbecke, distinguished guests, ladies and gentlemen,

There are three sponsors of this Symposium.

Dr Wolfgang Mayr, from the University of Vienna, where Karl Landsteiner started his career, was greatly interested in sponsoring this symposium to honor the great master. Dr Mayr is the head of the clinical division for blood group serology and president of this year's 26th ISBT meeting.

The umbrella organisation of the Viennese municipal hospitals, the "Wiener Krankenanstaltenverbund" with its managing director Dr Eugen Hauke as well as the responsible City Counsellor of Public Health and Hospitals, Dr Sepp Rieder, were also very interested in sponsoring this symposium in memory of Karl Landsteiner. It was while Landsteiner served as head of Pathology at the "Wilheminenspital", one of the leading hospitals of Vienna, that he made the landmark discovery that poliomyelitis can be transmitted from polio victims to monkeys.

The third sponsor is the Karl Landsteiner & Eisler-Terramare Foundation, inaugurated as a memorial foundation a few years ago. The objectives of this Foundation are to honor outstanding Austrian scientists in the field of immunology as well as to promote and foster the scientific endeavors of promising young Austrian immunologists.

During the early years of the 20th century, after the discovery of blood groups, Karl Landsteiner proceeded with his experiments on erythrocyte agglutination and lysis together with his younger colleague, Michael Eisler-Terramare. It is of interest to look more closely at the circumstances and aspirations of these two great Austrian immunologists. Each made discoveries in the years 1906 to 1908 that were milestones in the field of vaccine development.

Landsteiner's discovery that poliomyelitis can be transmitted from humans to monkeys opened the way; yet, it took half a century before the first formaldehyde inactivated polio vaccine could be applied to children. For the development of a safe and efficacious product, additional safety tests were needed. It is noteworthy that the crucial additional safety test applied was based on the observation Landsteiner had made in his first experiments: the transmission of the virus to monkeys.

Eisler-Terramare, on the other hand, succeeded, in cooperation with Loewenstein, in the detoxification of bacterial toxins while maintaining their immunologic structure. He was the first to start immunization in people with detoxified tetanus toxin. Alas, after the end of the First World War and the fall of the Austro-Hungarian empire, any scientific activity was seriously impaired in this part of the world. The discoveries of Eisler-Terramare and Loewenstein were taken up successfully by scientists in France and England, resulting in the large-scale manufacture of diphtheria and tetanus vaccines.

It is ironic that the basic desire of each of these scientists remained unfulfilled. Not even after having been awarded the Nobel Prize did Landsteiner's ambition to become head of a large scientific institution materialize. Eisler-Terramare's wish to be awarded the Nobel Prize for his important discovery, which had provided the basis for safe and efficacious vaccine preparations with formaldehyde inactivation of micro-organisms or their toxic products, did not come true. However, Eisler-Terramare was appointed scientific director of the Serotherapeutic Institute in Vienna. In the meantime, Landsteiner received the Nobel Prize for Medicine in 1930.

Karl Landsteiner left Austria with his family towards the end of 1919. He was scientifically active at the Rockefeller Institute until the end of his life and died in New York during the Second World War. Eisler-Terramare miraculously survived a Nazi concentration camp and was reappointed scientific director of the Serotherapeutic Institute, a position he held until his demise.

Landsteiner was the first to recognize that the bases of antigenic specificity are chemical structures he called determinants. He considered this discovery as his most important contribution to science, and he confessed to his friends and colleagues that he was rather disappointed at not being awarded the Nobel Prize for this new and fascinating area of immunology emerging from his studies, instead of a discovery made thirty years ago. The aim of this symposium is to highlight the scientific developments in the field of immunology concerning epitope recognition achieved since Landsteiner's discovery.

On behalf of the sponsors, it is my pleasure to welcome you to this symposium and to wish you a successful and most interesting meeting.

HANS EIBL

Preface

On July 16th 2000, a number of Immunologists assembled to commemorate the Nobel-prize winning work of Karl Landsteiner produced 100 years ago in Vienna, the City where this important scientist began several of his seminal contributions to Immunology. As stated by Dr. Hans Eibl in his welcoming address, a major aim of the symposium was to highlight the scientific developments in the field of Immunology concerning epitope recognition, since the discovery by Landsteiner of the importance of antibody recognition of specific chemical structures, "antigenic determinants". Several of the talks delivered at this symposium are published in this volume.

The first contribution is by Dr. Pauline Mazumdar, a specialist in the history of science and scholarly author of "*Species and Specificity: An Interpretation of the History of Immunology*". In her chapter here, she lucidly describes the scientific background in Vienna during Landsteiner's time and the relationship to his contemporary Immunologists, Paul Ehrlich in particular.

The intricate knowledge and insight of the next contributor, Dr. Herman Eisen, into the subject of antigenic specificity is truly impressive. Starting from Landsteiner's discovery of cross-reacting determinants, he brings the reader within a few pages across many decades of research in B and T cell specificity, emphasizing the heterogeneity of antibodies and the degeneracy in antigen recognition by T cells.

Dr. Jack Strominger and coworkers describe the use of an inventive method, involving oligomerization of antigenic epitopes of autoantigens, to specifically and effectively eliminate the responsiveness of epitope-specific T cells. In those cases where the major epitopes of autoantigens involved in an auto-immune disease are known, such an approach could be very useful.

Dr. Eli Sercarz provides an elegant excursion into the realm of T cell specificities and the complications that can arise during presentation to the T cell of individual peptides. He emphasizes the series of selections involved in arriving at the antigenic determinant representing the winning compromise recognized by the memory T cells in the evolved immune response.

The danger resulting from antigenic mimicry between bacterial and endogenous peptides is very beautifully illustrated by the report from Drs. Josef Penninger and Kurt Bachmaier, who show that cardiomyopathy can be the result of autoimmunity against a-myosin, triggered by the immune response against Chlamydia and a number of other pathogens.

Finally, Dr. Marion Scott reviews the history of the discovery of the Rh Blood Group system and the participation in this from Landsteiner and Wiener. She then briefly describes the current state of our knowledge concerning the mosaic of epitopes of the Rh D antigen and the relationship between the serological activity and the molecular biology of Rh D.

Landsteiner is best known for his discovery of the human blood groups. The revolutionary discoveries of this brilliant scientist in other fields have not received the recognition they deserve. His demonstration that poliomyelitis is transmissable showed the way for modern virology. His studies opening the field for epitope recognition, which he himself considered his main achievement, laid the foundation for research ongoing in our days. This meeting with its outstanding contributors is but a small tribute to this visionary scientist.

G. JEANETTE THORBECKE †
WOLFGANG R. MAYR
MARTHA M. EIBL

Contents

Contributors

AVENT, N. D.
Bristol Institute for Transfusion Sciences, Bristol
and
University of the West of England, Bristol,
UK

BACHMEIER, K.
Amgen Institute, Ontario Cancer Institute,
Department of Medical Biophysics, University of Toronto,
620 University Avenue, Suite 706, Toronto, Ontario M5G 2C1,
Canada

BEECH, J.
La Jolla Institute for Allergy and Immunology,
10355 Science Center Drive, San Diego, California 92121,
USA

BROSNAN, C.
Department of Pathology, Albert Einstein College of Medicine,
Bronx, New York 10461, USA

CAMPAGNONI, A.
La Jolla Institute for Allergy and Immunology,
10355 Science Center Drive, San Diego, California 92121,
USA

DENG, H.
La Jolla Institute for Allergy and Immunology,
10355 Science Center Drive, San Diego, California, 92121,
USA

DORF, M. E.
Department of Pathology, Harvard Medical School, Boston,
Massachusetts 02115,
USA

EISEN, H. N.
Center for Cancer Research and Department of Biology,
Massachusetts Institute of Technology, Cambridge,
Massachusetts, USA

ELZEN, P. VAN DEN
La Jolla Institute for Allergy and Immunology,
10355 Science Center Drive, San Diego, California, 92121,
USA

FALK, K.
Department of Molecular and Cellular Biology,
Harvard University, 7 Divinity Avenue, Cambridge, MA 02138,
USA

JONES, J. W.
Bristol Institute for Transfusion Sciences, Bristol
and
National Blood Service, Liverpool,
UK

KUMAR, V.
La Jolla Institute for Allergy and Immunology,
10355 Science Center Drive, San Diego, California, 92121,
USA

LIU, W.
Bristol Institute for Transfusion Sciences, Bristol
and
National Blood Service, Liverpool,
UK

MADAKAMUTIL, L. T.
La Jolla Institute for Allergy and Immunology,
10355 Science Center Drive, San Diego, California, 92121,
USA

MAVERAKIS, E.
La Jolla Institute for Allergy and Immunology,
10355 Science Center Drive, San Diego, California, 92121,
USA

MAZUMDAR, P. M. H.
Institute for History and Philosophy of Science
and Technology, Victoria College, University of Toronto,
91 Charles Street West, Toronto, Ontario M5S 1K7,
Canada

MOUDGIL, K.
La Jolla Institute for Allergy and Immunology,
10355 Science Center Drive, San Diego, California, 92121,
USA

PENNINGER, J. M.
Amgen Institute, Ontario Cancer Institute, Department of
Medical Biophysics, University of Toronto, 620 University Avenue, Suite 706, Toronto, Ontario M5G 2C1,
Canada

RIA, F.
La Jolla Institute for Allergy and Immunology,
10355 Science Center Drive, San Diego, California, 92121,
USA

RÖTZSCHKE, O.
Department of Molecular and Cellular Biology,
Harvard University, 7 Divinity Avenue, Cambridge, MA 02138,
USA

SANTAMBROGIO, L.
Department of Cancer Immunology and AIDS,
Dana-Farber Cancer Institute, Boston, Massachusetts, 02115,
USA

SCHNEIDER, S. C.
La Jolla Institute for Allergy and Immunology,
10355 Science Center Drive, San Diego, California, 92121,
USA

SCOTT, M. L.
    Bristol Institute for Transfusion Sciences, Bristol,
    UK

SERCARZ, E. E.
    La Jolla Institute for Allergy and Immunology,
    10355 Science Center Drive, San Diego, California, 92121,
    USA

STROMINGER, J. L.
    Department of Molecular and Cellular Biology,
    Harvard University, 7 Divinity Avenue, Cambridge, MA 02138
    and
    Department of Cancer Immunology and AIDS,
    Dana-Farber Cancer Institute, Boston, MA 02115,
    USA

VOAK, D.
    National Blood Service, Cambridge,
    UK

CHAPTER 1

Landsteiner In Vienna

P. M. H. Mazumdar[1]

We are here today to celebrate Karl Landsteiner and his work, and how it seems one hundred years later. That's odd, really. Landsteiner himself would never have expected it; he was a man who never felt he was a success. Well educated in the best laboratories of his time, enormously hard working and productive, he left Vienna in 1919, when he realised that he would never get his chair, and never direct his own institute.

Landsteiner was born in 1868, in Baden bei Wien, just outside the city. The Vienna of his early years was a remarkable city of culture. Art, music, literature, architecture and science all flourished in the period stretching from the late XIXth to the early XXth century. His father, Leopold Landsteiner, was a political and economic journalist and newspaper editor, a member of the cultured Jewish elite, but he died in 1875, when his son was only six [1] (Fig. 1).

From then on, Karl Landsteiner was brought up by his mother. She was from Prossnitz in Moravia, from a Jewish merchant family, and she was twenty years younger than Leopold. They had been married for only seven years when she was widowed. She and her son were very close: after she died in 1908, Karl Landsteiner kept her picture with him for the rest of his life. (Fig. 2)

Instead of reading law, like most of the students from his father's intellectual background, Landsteiner chose the Vienna Medical School. There were Jews in the Medical School, but there was also anti-Semitism among the students. Jews were not generally allowed to join the student societies, but there was a Jewish one; Landsteiner may have belonged to it – he had a scar on his face in the approved manner [2]. Jewish teachers were not eligible for the higher university posts, unless they converted. Professorships like other government jobs in the Austro-Hungarian Empire were open only to Catholics: strictly speaking, this policy was pro-Catholic, rather than anti-Semitic, though that probably did not make it any less painful for its victims. Many young people who aspired to a

[1] Institute for the History and Philosophy of Science and Technology, Victoria College, 73 Queen's Park Cresent East, University of Toronto, Toronto, Ontario M5S 1K7, Canada

Fig. 1. Karl Landsteiner at the age of about five, c. 1873. (Photograph from George Mackenzie's collection, courtesy of the American Philosophical Society, Philadelphia.)

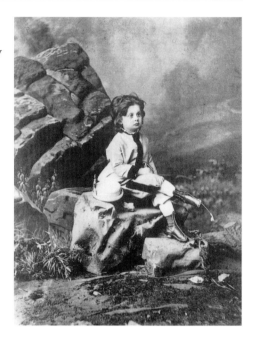

Fig. 2. Franziska (Fanni) Hess, Mrs Leopold Landsteiner, Karl's mother. (Photograph from George Mackenzie's collection, courtesy of the American Philosophical Society, Philadelphia.)

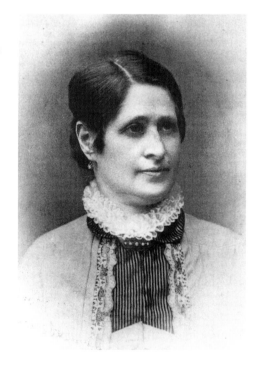

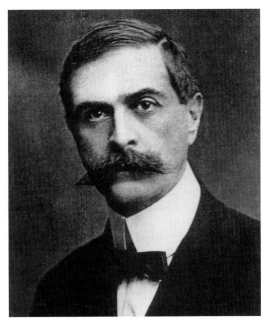

Fig. 3. Karl Landsteiner as a young man, c.1896. (Photograph from George Mackenzie's collection, courtesy of the American Philosophical Society, Philadelphia.)

serious academic career converted, and they seem to have been successfully assimilated [3]. Landsteiner and his mother converted in 1890, just before his final examination.

His first job was as Second Assistant to Max von Gruber at the Institute for Hygiene. He stayed in it just under two years, from January 1896 to September 1897, but I think it determined his point of view for the rest of his life. (Fig. 3)

As soon as he joined Gruber, Landsteiner became involved in Gruber's row with Paul Ehrlich. Ehrlich was director of the Frankfurt Royal Institute for Experimental Therapy – the serum institute – and by far the most important figure in the immunology of his day. His *Seitenkettentheorie* or side-chain theory, and the diagrams he used to symbolise it, seemed to explain everything that one needed to know about antigen recognition and antibody formation. (Fig. 4) The symbols represented side-chains like those on a benzene ring, and imply a perfect one-to-one antigen-antibody specificity with a tight irreversible linkage, like the linkages of organic chemistry. To use the image made famous by the organic chemist Emil Fischer, they fitted each other like a lock and key.

Gruber, on the other hand, postulated a much looser, more quantitative idea of specificity: he saw it as a matter of *quantitative Abstufung*; an antibody reacted best with the antigen used to raise it, but slightly less well with a whole series of related antigens – stepwise, not sharply defined, specificity. He had

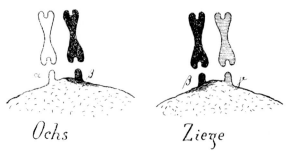

Fig. 4. Paul Ehrlich's theory of immunity symbolised. A rabbit anti-ox serum lyses both ox and goat cells; absorption with ox cells removes both reactions, but absorption with goat only removes the anti-goat effect. He suggests that ox and goat cells each have one unique, specific receptor and one receptor in common. This technique and this interpretation became the basis for blood-group studies from 1920 onwards. From Paul Ehrlich and Julius Morgenroth, "Über Hämolysine: sexte Mittheilung", *Berl. klin. Wschr.* (1901) 38 569–574; 598–604 (p. 570)

some angry exchanges at meetings about this with Ehrlich supporters. Gruber bad-mouthed Ehrlich publicly and often, and wittily. But Ehrlich and his theory were too well entrenched, and the leaders of the field, people like Richard Paltauf, Director of the Institute for Experimental Pathology and of the State Serum Institute in Vienna, were against Gruber. He couldn't win. In 1902, he accepted the chair of Hygiene in Munich.

When Landsteiner joined Gruber's laboratory, he was set to work on an experiment designed to support Gruber's idea of specificity: he was to test an immune serum against a group of bacterial species related to the species used to raise it. He came up with this statement:

> This then is specificity ... the phenomenon appears in traces with different species, but never as intensely as when matching (*gleichnamig*) serum and bacteria act on each other [4].

Now it may seem rather remarkable that he came to that very Gruberly conclusion. During the course of his medical training, Landsteiner had done the rounds of three of the most important chemical laboratories of his day. They were all organic chemists, interested in chemical structure, covalent linkages (to be a bit anachronistic) and organic syntheses, including synthetic arguments based on the placing of side-chains. You might have thought that Ehrlich's side-chain theory would have appealed to him. But one of these laboratories was Emil Fischer's, where he was working on the structure of the sugars, and where Fischer was to make his famous statement about the lock and key, in this case about the fermentation of different sugars by yeasts.

Fischer's series of natural and synthetic sugars differed from each other by small structural modifications, and his yeasts acted on them with stepwise, quantitatively different effects. (Fig. 5) Fischer's own use of the lock and key

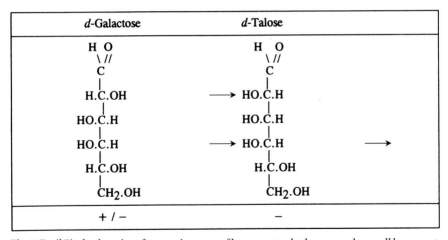

Fig. 5. Emil Fischer's series of stereo-isomers of hexose, attacked more-or-less well by a yeast. The top row have all the same three asymmetric C-atoms; the bottom left has one different, and the bottom right two. Modified from Emil Fischer, "Bedeutung der Stereochemie für die Physiologie", *Z. f. physiol. Chem.* (1898) 26 60–87; and Fischer and Hans Thierfelder, "Verhalten der verschiedenen Zucker gegen reine Hefen", *Ber. d. deut. chem. Ges.* (1894) 27 2031–2037.

analogy allowed for master keys that opened up several molecules more-or-less well. Ehrlich used the image to imply a multitude of different keys, each opening only one lock. Landsteiner never used the lock-and-key image – that had been appropriated by Ehrlich – but he did use Emil Fischer's idea of an organic series attacked more-or-less well by a ferment, and like Fischer, he scored the quantitative effect as +++ / ++ / + / +– and –. Fischer may also have provided him with a role model that he tried hard to emulate: that of the distant, dominant *Geheimrat*, the single all-powerful figure directing his own institute.

In 1899, he had already moved on to a post as Assistant in the Institute for Pathological Anatomy under Anton Weichselbaum, where he stayed until 1908. Here again, he took up a Gruber problem: he was still expanding on Gruber's idea that even dead bacteria would raise an immune response, showing that immunity was not just a protective reaction, but a more general feature of living organisms. Landsteiner broadened that idea to the raising of antibodies against completely harmless saprophytes, and against red blood cells. Gruber was very pleased with Landsteiner's conclusion. He felt that his own idea had been handed back to him in a more developed form, that of a general biological law uniting multifarious experience.

His work on the agglutination and lysis of red blood cells appeared in 1900. Most workers who had come across antibodies in human serum connected them with some disease or other. Landsteiner first suggested that they might be due to bacterial damage, or to some disease, which was the usual view of serum antibodies in general. Or perhaps, he said rather uncertainly, they *might* be related to individual differences. He admitted that they seemed specially strong in sera from seriously ill patients [5]. In 1901, he came out with the paper that explained the isoagglutinins in human blood in a way that cut through the tangle of supposed protective functions that had grown up around these mysterious antibodies [6]. They had no connection with disease: they were not related to typhoid or malaria, but to red cell antigens – including those of himself and his assistant, Adriano Sturli, a student at the Second Medical Clinic. He called the red cell antigens A, B, and C, and the antibodies anti-A and anti-B. A serum typically contained either anti-A or anti-B or both; no antibody was ever present that reacted with the subject's own cells, which could have A or B or neither, which would make it group C.

I sometimes feel that the clear-cut specificity of this was rather difficult for Landsteiner. It did not really conform to his *quantitative Abstufung*, or more-or-less good fit. And he did not follow it up for many years, long after he had left Vienna, though he was usually very sharp on matters of intellectual property: he let Sturli and one of Sturli's colleagues go on with the project, and they discovered the fourth blood group AB, which they called "without type", since it had no agglutinins in the serum [7]. In fact, this did seem more like an

Ehrlichean result. Ehrlich had been doing experiments in which he immunised a group of goats with each other's blood, and found that they would all produce several different specific antibodies. This was the first suggestion of immunological differences in the bloods of individuals of the same species, and Ehrlich and his co-worker Julius Morgenroth called it the pluralistic conception of immunity: the cells had many different receptors – Ehrlich's term –, and the immunised animal could produce a whole army, *eine ganze Schar*, of different specific immune bodies [8]. It was the kind of thing that Landsteiner felt explained nothing about immunity. There must be some unifying law that covered the whole series of phenomena. Simply postulating innumerable different substances, one for each effect, was "uneconomical". It was no simpler than the phenomena themselves. It could not be called an explanation at all. He speculated that seeming specificity was an additive effect, a combination of a series of substances non-specific in themselves [9].

He found the ideal additive effect in the new science of colloid chemistry, the physical chemistry of very large molecules – particles, even – which reacted reversibly with each other through surface charge, not, as in Ehrlich's theory, through side-chains and the firm bindings of organic chemistry. But he emphasised that the difference between a physical and a chemical compound itself is gradual and stepwise: the reactions of antigens and antibodies are influenced by chemical constitution, but in their quantitative relations they are like physical phenomena, such as solubility. The mutual precipitation of charged colloids was a model of the antigen-antibody reaction, but without the specificity. It provided a prediction that could be tested.

Landsteiner's supporter in this was the colloid chemist Wolfgang Pauli, one year older than Landsteiner. His interest was in the properties of colloids that were important in physiology – in fact, he felt that colloids were the stuff of life, and the new electrochemistry gave a unique insight into life itself. The proteins could not be analysed by the methods of ordinary chemistry: they did not conform to the law of definite proportions. Life processes belonged to a different universe, whose laws were the laws of colloid chemistry, where the reactions often conformed to no fixed proportions. In immunology, this was a point of view that had a good deal of attractiveness. As Jules Bordet said in 1903, it had been argued that antigen and antibody must combine in definite proportions because twice as much serum is needed to combine with twice the dose of antigen; he thought that was as reasonable as claiming that paint must combine in definite proportions with a wall [10].

These ideas were very attractive to Landsteiner. They bore out his intuitive feeling that specificity was not absolute but quantitative and stepwise, and his feeling that an explanation must be general and unifying, not pluralistic like Ehrlich's. They exactly reflected his theory of scientific knowledge, which he laid out at length in a paper of 1909 – the year after Ehrlich was awarded his Nobel Prize. In it he criticized Ehrlich's theory and compared it with his own, in which a few substances of low specificity combined to make many more highly specific ones:

> According to the older view, for every single effect of a serum, there was a separate substance, or at least a particular chemical group ... The situation was undoubtedly made much simpler if , to use the Ehrlich terminology, ... the separate haptophore groups can combine with an extremely large number of receptors in stepwise differing quantities ... A normal serum would therefore visibly affect such a large number of different blood cells ... not because it contained countless special substances, but because of the colloids of the serum, and therefore of the agglutinins by reason of their chemical constitution and the electrochemical properties resulting from it. That this view represents a considerable simplification is clear. It also opens the way to direct experimental testing by the methods of structural chemistry [11].

He goes on to say that this sounds like it is only an analogy, but analogies are one of the most important means to knowledge. With this colloid-chemical view, you can imitate agglutination with simple substances – the analogy leads to a simple model that can be used to test the hypothesis. In short, he is saying that a hypothesis must make the phenomena simpler to understand; it must unite the diverse phenomena with each other by continuous stepwise differences. Unity, simplicity and continuity – those are his key words.

I have often wondered whether Landsteiner had any contact with the philosopher Ernst Mach, whose philosophy of science sounds very much like this. Mach had had the chair of philosophy in Vienna since 1895 – he died in 1916 – and his popular lectures were a runaway success. As Janik and Toulmin said in 1973, seldom has a scientist exerted such an influence upon his culture as has Ernst Mach [12]. His essay on economy of thought was particularly well known and often reprinted. Economy and simplicity are the essence of what science does – every scientific law is a general expression of the relation of facts to each other in a more economical way, a continuous, quantitative way if possible. Mach was very close to Wolfgang Pauli, and Landsteiner might have met him. But you wouldn't need to meet him to know what he was saying – his "economy and simplicity" were all over the cultured world of Vienna, and they were applied as much to architectural style, and even music, as they were to science [13].

The colloid analogy excited Landsteiner. In January 1904, he had sent off a short, speculative paper to the Vienna medical weekly on the analogy between the mutual precipitation of charged colloids and serological precipitation [14]. That was probably to secure priority for the concept. When the Vienna colloid chemist Jean Billitzer took up the idea in 1905, in the *Zeitschrift für physikalische Chemie*, and did not refer to him, he wrote a sharp note to the journal pointing out his priority. It obviously meant more to him than the apparently sharp specificity of the blood groups. Pauli lost no opportunity for praising and publicising Landsteiner's work, and together they developed an apparatus for determining the charge of proteins and other colloids, and they presented it at the 1908 meeting of the Congress for Internal Medicine [15]. Their suggestion was that heavily charged colloids like silica gel would naturally just precipitate anything, but more subtly charged amphoteric molecules like the proteins might be the bearers of specificity. A later version of this moving boundary electrophoresis apparatus was adopted by Leonor Michaelis of Berlin, and then in 1930 by the Swedish physical chemist Arne Tiselius; it is usually known as a Tiselius apparatus nowadays.

In 1908, Landsteiner moved on to the department of Pathology at the Wilhelminen Hospital. It was rather unusual to have a pathologist very deeply involved in research: they were mostly too busy with hospital post-mortems, histology and so on, and it generally wasn't regarded as an academic post. But he made time for his work with Pauli, as well as other projects, some of them coming out of his hospital work. This was a man of extraordinary productivity. One of Landsteiner's projects was on the specificity of the Wassermann reaction, the serological test for syphilis. He and his two co-workers claimed that it was not a specific reaction between a syphilitic antigen and antibody as Wassermann himself supposed when he introduced it in 1906 [16]. It could be carried out with substitute antigens such as lipids and alcoholised beef heart, and Landsteiner interpreted it as a non-specific colloidal reaction [17]. His co-worker Rudolf Müller went on to work out a simplified colloidal version of the test that he hoped would replace the original Wassermann as a diagnostic tool [18].

This view did not impress the immunological establishment, represented in Vienna by Richard Paltauf and his group. Erna Lesky calls Paltauf "one of the great school-builders" of the Vienna Medical School [19]. In 1893, he had started the State Serum Institute and in 1900, he was appointed Professor and Director of the Institute for Pathology as well. He and his people were supporters of the Ehrlich school of thought, and bitter opponents of Max von Gruber. The bread and butter of a serum institute was the production and standardisation of antisera for therapy and for bacteriological identification, according to the standardisation method worked out by Paul Ehrlich and adopted by serum institutes world-wide. A theory that did not give full weight to a sharply defined specificity would seem to a practical serologist to be self-defeating: as Richard

Volk of the State Serum Institute said, "If agglutination is to be used as a tool for the diagnosis of either disease or bacteria, the first and most important requirement is that the specificity of the reaction must be postulated" [20]. More-or-less-good fit was not much use in identifying bacteria.

Vienna was an immunological scene that was fertile in new ideas. Landsteiner had adopted the point of view of his first mentor, Max von Gruber. Then he had linked up with Wolfgang Pauli, the colloid chemist. Now he found a new source of inspiration in the work of Ernst Peter Pick, a young man who had started at the Serum Institute in 1899 under Paltauf, and then in 1906, moved over to the Institute for Pharmacology. Pick's work at the Serum Institute shows the stamp of an Ehrlich team player. He and his colleague Friedrich Obermeyer introduced a diazo-group into serum albumins from several different species, and used it to link other groups to the proteins. With the introduction of the new groups, the original species specificity completely disappeared. An antiserum raised against iodo-diazo-albumin from any animal reacted with an iodo-diazo-albumin from any other [21]. To someone based in Paltauf's Institute, this looked like a perfect justification for Ehrlich's side-chain theory of immunity. The determinant might be literally a side-chain of a benzene ring, perhaps the ring in the amino-acid tyrosine. But soon after this came out, Pick left the Serum Institute. And when he wrote a long review paper the following year, he had abandoned the side-chain theory:

> The only thing we know about the physico-chemical nature of antigens ... is that they are colloids. In our opinion, nothing prevents us regarding the production of antibodies by antigens as the result of the formation of adsorption complexes between certain colloids and the toxins. A similar conception of the effect of toxin on antitoxin has gradually gained ground through the investigations of Landsteiner and Biltz (see also Pauli ...) [22].

It seems that as soon as Pick left the Serum Institute, he threw off the Ehrlich yoke and went over to colloids. Here he sets up an alternative to both Ehrlich's conception of antibody production, and his covalent-binding view of the antigen-antibody reaction. Landsteiner took it up, suggesting that:

> Immune chemistry is the chemistry of the amphoteric colloids. But this is not an explanation of specificity as the theory of the influence of amphoteric colloids is not fully worked out. ... Acidic or basic groups may be important in the fine adjustment of their electrical behaviour ... [23].

Colloid is the key word: it is not an explanation in itself, but it allows the tight bindings of organic chemistry to be replaced by a reversible, quantitative and

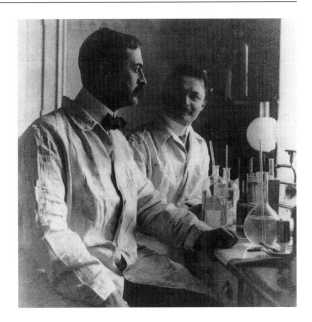

Fig. 6. Landsteiner and his co-worker Emil Prášek from Belgrade, photo d. 14 December 1913. (Photograph from George Mackenzie's collection, courtesy of the American Philosophical Society, Philadelphia.)

stepwise conception of specificity. Electrical behaviour, acidity and basicity and chemical constitution can all be drawn together to define an antigen.

In 1913, with the help of Emil Prášek, Landsteiner started on the series of experiments to investigate the nature of antigenicity. (Fig. 6) Landsteiner and Prášek began by repeating all of Obermeyer and Pick's work, and re-interpreting it. And in place of Obermeyer and Pick's conclusion that species specificity had vanished at a stroke when they inserted the side-chains, Landsteiner and Prášek found that there was a graduated stepwise effect: the three anti-horse nitro-albumin sera they had made still reacted better with the horse nitro-albumin than with bovine or chicken nitro-albumins, and they still reacted weakly with the native horse albumin [24].

The next step was to change the charge of the albumins: they alkylated the protein, blocking its acid groups to form esters. Technically, these experiments were very difficult. Sometimes the substitutions did not work. When they did, the treated albumin was insoluble, and it was difficult to get a good response to it. They could not use a precipitin test, because the substance was already precipitated, so they had to use complement binding, notoriously cumbersome and clumsy. But the results were clear – only the charged groups were involved in ester formation, and Landsteiner concluded that all was stepwise: as the species specificity diminished, the new specificity increased. When the species specificity was quite gone, the treated albumin had become antigenic in its species of origin.

The immunology was clear, but the exact structure of the antigenic material was not. With a new co-worker, Hans Lampl, he started a new lot of experiments to link the immunology with the position of the charged substituents. It was an immense effort: hundreds of compounds were synthesized and tested and hundreds of animals were immunised. It is a very long paper, with a long and unsatisfactory conclusion [25]. They still did not know what the structure of the test substances was. These experiments were going on during the first World War. It was very difficult to work in Vienna: Landsteiner mentions that the animals didn't give a good response because they were not fed enough, and there was no heating. The workers, too, were famished and frozen; they tried to keep going as the city collapsed and the Empire crumbled around them.

Then in 1917, they came across a new method for inserting diazo-compounds which showed that the tyrosine ring of the protein took on two diazo groups and formed a bis-diazo-tyrosine. Bis-diazo-tyrosine was a known quantity, that could be substituted in known ways. It could even be made soluble. They made up a series of variants on diazo-benzene sulphonate, and attached them to horse albumin – 33 different antigens, 23 sera and 759 test reactions – an enormous project, carried out under the most difficult circumstances, but finally coming out to the hoped-for result [26] (Fig. 7).

With this paper, Landsteiner answered the questions of 1896 in a way that Max von Gruber would have approved. There were no absolute, clear-cut differences in specificity, only stepwise gradations in intensity. He includes the idea of charge – it's the charged groups that matter – from his Pauli days, and the idea of chemical structure, from his Pick days, and from the model of the action of yeast on the sugar series, from Fischer. He knew he had reached his goal, the definition of specificity as smoothly graded differences. This was the proof that he had been struggling towards for about 25 years, from his earliest days in immunology. It conformed to his philosophy of scientific knowledge, as well as solving a scientific problem.

By 1919, Landsteiner was 51, and had published 171 papers, many of them of the highest rank. But although he was so productive, he had not had a good career in Vienna. He had seen his colleagues promoted past him, getting their professorships and directorships before the War, while he remained at the Wilhelminen Hospital doing post-mortems. He had been appointed Associate Professor in 1911. In 1919, Wolfgang Pauli got his professorship and became Director of the Institute for Colloid Chemistry. Landsteiner felt keenly that *he* should have been appreciated more highly, and perhaps that he should have been in line for the succession to Paltauf. Why was he not? It is difficult to be sure, because Landsteiner himself would not talk about his Vienna period,

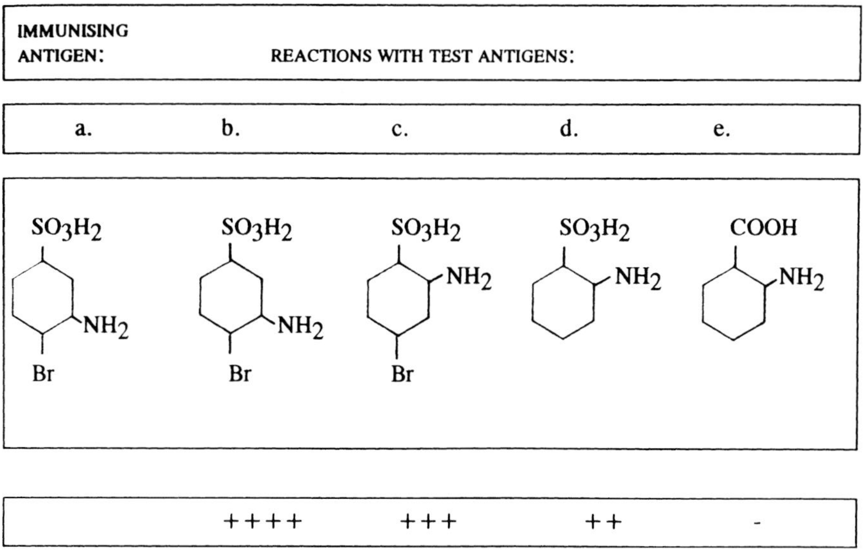

IMMUNISING ANTIGEN:	REACTIONS WITH TEST ANTIGENS:			
a.	b.	c.	d.	e.
SO_3H_2 ... NH_2 ... Br	SO_3H_2 ... NH_2 ... Br	SO_3H_2 ... NH_2 ... Br	SO_3H_2 ... NH_2	$COOH$ ... NH_2
	++++	+++	++	-

Fig. 7. Chemical structure and immune specificity: demonstration by Landsteiner and Hans Lampl, showing a continuous spectrum of reactions to the benzene-sulphonic acid family of antigens. The serum raised against a. gives its strongest reaction with b, the identical substance. It also reacts but more weakly with c, more weakly still with d. and not at all with e. Landsteiner feels that this cannot be explained by "innumerable different antibodies" with single sharp specificities à la Ehrlich, but by specificity which consists of more-or-less good fit between antibody and a series of antigens. The experiment and the quantitative scoring recall Fischer's sugar experiment (see Fig. 5.) From Landsteiner and Lampl, "Über die Antigeneigenschaften von Azoprotein: XI Mitteilung über Antigene", *Z. f. Immunitätsforschung* (1917) 26 293–304 (p. 343).

although it seems to me that it was the most important and the most productive period of his life, and the most fertile environment that he could have found to work in, at least up till the beginning of the War.

One possible reason could have been anti-Semitism. The *Ordinarius* or Full Professorship, could not be held by a practising Jew, but many people simply converted and usually got their posting: the Landsteiners had converted about thirty years earlier. Max von Gruber was Jewish, as were E.P. Pick and Wolfgang Pauli, who got his Directorship in 1919. There certainly was a growing strain of anti-Semitism following the end of the War, but according to Pick, it did not affect Landsteiner personally [27]. Pick felt that Landsteiner was afraid of the future in post-war Vienna, rather than of anti-Semitism. He got married in 1916 to Helene Wlasto, a member of the Greek Orthodox Church, who converted to Catholicism soon afterwards. They now had a son, and life in Vienna as the state and the monarchy foundered after the end of the war was very hard. The Polish immunologist Ludwik Hirszfeld who visited at the end of 1918, said that Landsteiner had been a handsome, upright man. But now he looked as if he was starving [28].

Max von Gruber, Landsteiner's old mentor, thought he knew why Landsteiner had never been promoted. It was because he had set himself up against Ehrlich – a position that had led to Gruber himself leaving Vienna in 1902. Even in 1919, Ehrlich's theory of immunity was not dead. It could not be killed off by a simple publication of results. Ehrlich had never tried to specify what exactly his so-called receptors were, only that they differed sharply from each other. His suggestion of a "chemical union" between antigen and antibody was a metaphor, rather like his Fischerian "lock and key." The receptors remained at the level of a heuristic diagram, a diagram that has been extraordinarily persistent in immunology. His point of view was deeply entrenched wherever sharp specificity was important in practice, especially in the serum institutes. Landsteiner's ideas did not have a practical value in that setting, where nobody wanted a matter of more-or-less good fit. He was a marginal man in the world of German-speaking immunology. In addition, investigation of the chemical basis of immunity in itself was becoming increasingly unfashionable. The Ehrlich group had simply stopped discussing it. He was never going to get his professorship, nor was he going to succeed Paltauf: that was to go to one of Paltauf's men. In the face of all this, the conversion to Catholicism that had been enough for others did not help him.

Landsteiner had been very loyal to the Austro-Hungarian monarchy; he had been awarded the title of *Regierungsrat* during the War, in recognition of his service at the No. 1 Military Hospital. He never forgot that loyalty, though he took the oath to the new republican régime in 1919 [29]. But his life in Vienna was too difficult and too personally problematic. In 1919, he got an appointment as pathologist at the R.K. Ziekenhaus, a general hospital in The Hague in Holland. On 27 May 1920, he resigned from the Wilhelminen Hospital and took his pension. Like Gruber, he left Vienna for good. It was a hard decision.

This story has something of a happy ending, as you know. Landsteiner was contacted by Simon Flexner, Director of the Rockefeller Institute in New York, and in 1922, he left Europe for the US. In New York, he pursued both the work on blood groups and on the charge outline of chemically defined antigens for another 20 years with great success. In 1930, he was awarded the Nobel Prize for his discovery of the ABO blood groups. But Landsteiner was not a man to allow himself to be happy. He had been made head of a department at the Rockefeller, but he was never to be Director of his own institute. And he always felt that he should have got the prize for his work on antigens, not for the blood groups.

Acknowledgement

My thanks to the participants of the Landsteiner Symposium for good questions and other contributions.

References

1. Rudolf Till, "Erhebungen durch Archiverei der Gemeinde Wien", material gathered at the request of George Mackenzie, 1949–1951; American Philosophical Society, Landsteiner-Mackenzie Papers, B L32m, Box 2.
2. I am told that the student fraternity "Kadimah" founded in 1882 accepted only Jews.
3. Steven Beller, Vienna and the Jews, 1867–1938: a Cultural History (Cambridge: Cambridge University Press, 1989) 43–70
4. Karl Landsteiner (1897) "Über die Folgen der Einverleibung sterilisierter Bakterienkulturen", Wiener klin Wschr 10:439–444 (442)
5. Karl Landsteiner (1900) "Zur Kenntnis der antifermentativen, lytischen und agglutinierenden Wirkungen des Blutserums und der Lymphe", Zbl f Bakt 27:357–362 (fn.1); P.M.H. Mazumdar, "The purpose of immunity: Landsteiner's explanation of the human isoantibodies", J Hist Biol (1975) 8 115–134; Peter Keating, "The problem of natural antibodies, 1894–1905", J Hist Biol (1991) 24 245–263
6. Karl Landsteiner(1901) "Über Aggluninationserscheinungen normalen menschlichen Blutes", Wiener klin Wschr 14:1132–1134
7. Alfred von Decastello-Rechtwehr, Adriano Sturli (1902) "Über die Isoagglutinin im Serum gesunder und kranker Menschen", Münchener med Wschr 1090–1095
8. Paul Ehrlich, Julius Morgenroth (1900) "Über Hämolysine: dritte Mittheilung", Berl klin Wschr 37:453–458
9. Karl Landsteiner, Adriano Sturli (1902) "Hämagglutinine normaler Sera", Wiener klin Wschr 38–40; Karl Landsteiner, "Über Serumagglutinine", Münchener med Wschr (1902) 49:1905–1908
10. Jules Bordet (1903) "Sur le mode d'action des antitoxines sur les toxines", Ann. de l'Inst. Pasteur 17:161-186
11. Karl Landsteiner (1909) "Die Theorien der Antikörperbildung", Wiener klin Wschr 22:1623–1631 (p. 15)
12. Allan Janik, Stephen Toulmin (1973) Wittgenstein's Vienna (New York, NY: Simon & Schuster) 133–135
13. For further discussion of Landsteiner's philosophy of science and its the possible connection with Mach's, see Pauline M. H. Mazumdar, Species and specificity: an interpretation of the history of immunology (Cambridge, Cambridge University Press, 1995) 147–151; 152–175.
14. Karl Landsteiner, Nikolaus von Jagic (1904) "Über Analogien der Wirkung kolloidaler Kieselsäure mit der Reaction der Immunkörper und verwandter Stoffe", Wiener klin. Wschr. 17:63–64
15. Karl Landsteiner, Wolfgang Pauli, "Elektrische Wanderung der Immunstoffe", Verh d Kongr f inn Med (XX Congress, Vienna 1908) 571–574

16. August Wassermann, Max Neisser, Carl Brück (1906) "Eine serodiagnostische Reaktion bei Syphilis", Deutsche med Wschr 32:745

17. Karl Landsteiner, Rudolf Müller, Otto Pötzl (1907) "Über Komplimentbindungs-reaktionen bei Syphilis", Wiener klin Wschr 20:1565–1567

18. Rudolf Müller (1926) "Ballungsreaktion (Conglobation) mit luetischen Seris", Archiv f Dermat 151:570–578. In 1918, Müller was appointed head of the serodiagnostic depart-ment of the Wiener Allgemeines Krankenhaus. He did not join the Serum Institute. See Helmuth Gröger, "Karl Landsteiner and medical science in Vienna around 1900. The significance of laboratory medicine for clinical medicine", Vox Sanguinis (2000) 78 (suppl. 2) 003-006; Pauline M. H. Mazumdar, "The League of Nations standardises syphilis tests", in press (2000)

19. Erna Lesky, Die Wiener medizinische Schule im XIX Jahrhundert (Graz: Böhlaus, 1965) 577–578

20. Richard Volk, "Antikörper zu diagnostischen Zwecken (Serodiagnostik): über Aggluti-nation", in Rudolf Kraus and Constantin Levaditi, Handbuch der Technik und Methodik der Immunitätsforschung 2v in 3 (Jena: Fischer, 1st ed., 1908–1913) v2 Antikörper, 621–689 (664)

21. Friedrich Obermeyer, Ernst Peter Pick (1906) "Über die chemischen Grundlagen der Arteigenschaften der Eiweisskörper. Bildung von Immunpräcipitinen durch chemische veränderte Eiweisskörper", Wiener klin Wschr 19:327–333

22. Pick EP "Darstellung der Antigene mit chemischen und physikalischen Methoden", in Rudolf Kraus and Constantin Levaditi, eds, Handbuch der Technik und Methodik der Immunitätsforschung 2v (Jena: Fischer, 1908) v 1: Antigene 331–586 (p. 332)

23. Karl Landsteiner (1909) "Die Theorien der Antikörperbildung", Wiener klin Wschr 22:1623–1631

24. Karl Landsteiner, Emil Prásek (1913) "Über die Aufhebung der Artspezifizität von Serumeiweiss: IV Mitteilung über Antigene", Z f Immunitätsf 20:211–237

25. Karl Landsteiner, Hans Lampl (1917) "Über Antigene mit verschiedenartigen Acyl-gruppen: X Mitteilung über Antigene", Z f Immunitätsf 26:258–276

26. Karl Landsteiner, Hans Lampl (1917) "Über die Antigeneigenschaften von Azoprotein: XI Mitteilung über Antigene", Z f Immunitätsf 26:293–304

27. Pick EP, ltr to George Mackenzie d. 28 Feb 1949.Mackenzie Papers, B L23m, Box 2, Am Phil Soc

28. Ludwik Hirszfeld, Historia Zednego Zycia Hanna Hirszfeld, ed., (Warsaw: Institut Wydawniczy Pax, 1957) ms transl. 67

29. Paul Speiser, Ferdinand G. Smekal, Karl Landsteiner, the Discoverer of the Human Blood Groups and a Pioneer in the Field of Immunology. Biography of a Nobel Prize-Winner of the Vienna Medical School transl. Richard Rickett (Vienna: Gebr. Hollinek, 1975) 54, 57

CHAPTER 2

Antigen Recognition: 100 Years After Landsteiner

H. N. Eisen[1]

A central feature of the adaptive immune system is its capacity to distinguish among an immense number of different structures. The efforts made over the past century to understand this extraordinary ability grew largely from Landsteiner's work on the reactions of antisera with the small organic molecules he called haptens, or partial antigens, to indicate that they could react specifically with antibodies but not elicit antibody production. It was only near the end of his long, productive life that it became clear (through the work of Heidelberger and colleagues with polysaccharide antigens) that antibodies are proteins. And it was not until a few years after his death in 1943 that proteins were shown, by Fred Sanger, to be authentic molecules (rather than colloids) composed of linear chains of amino acids joined in α peptide bonds. It is thus understandable that in Landsteiner's monumental monograph on *The Specificity of Serological Reactions* he cautiously attributed the specificity of antisera to "...*the disproportional action of a number of similar agents on a variety of related substrata*" (1). By agents, he meant antibodies, of course, and by substrata he meant antigens or haptens. Today, having the benefit of over 60 years of further intensive study in many laboratories we can define specificity simply and more clearly as the ability "...to bind one unique chemical structure more strongly than a number of similar alternatives" (2).

Diversity of Antibodies to a Haptenic Group

Landsteiner's work dispelled any notion that might have once been held that there is absolute specificity in immune reactions. Indeed, the structures of the many cross-reacting molecules uncovered in work from his laboratory were used to great advantage to illuminate how a ligand's shape, size, and charge

[1] Center for Cancer Research and Department of Biology, Massachusetts Institute of Technology, Cambridge, Massachusetts, USA.

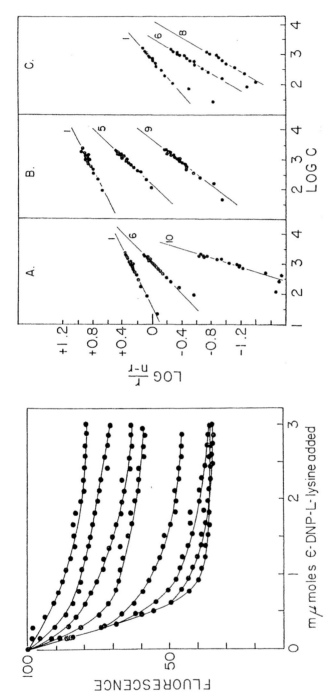

Fig. 1. Diversity of antibodies to the 2,4-dinitrophenyl (DNP) group produced in a rabbit against a DNP-protein conjugate. **A.** (left) The binding of ε-DNP lysine to sequentially precipitated sets of antibodies is revealed by quenching of the antibodies' tryptophan fluorescence. **B.** (right) The data of selected antibody sets in panel A is plotted according to the Sips distribution (logarithmic form) to reveal heterogeneity with regard to equilibrium constant (slope < 1.0.). From ref. 3

distribution affects the extent to which it is recognized by antibodies. He would not have been at all surprised by the data shown in Fig. 1. The Figure shows that in serum from rabbits immunized with a 2,4-dinitrophenyl-protein conjugate, the antibodies to the 2,4-dinitrophenyl (DNP) group can be subdivided into many subsets (3). The subsets were obtained by precipitating them serially by sequential additions of small amounts of a DNP-protein and then isolating the precipitated antibody and examining its binding of ε-DNP-lysine, a representative of the principal epitope in the immunizing protein conjugate. Increasing concentrations of ε-DNP-lysine (the ligand) led to increasing occupancy of antibody binding sites, as revealed by increasing quenching of the antibody's tryptophan fluorescence (Fig. 1A). The titration yields the average affinity (equilibrium constant) for the ligand of the antibody molecules in each subset. It is obvious that the first precipitated set of antibodies had the highest average affinity and that successive ones had progressively lower average affinities. The titration also made it possible to estimate the degree of binding constant heterogeneity in each sample (Fig. 1B). Not only was the total population heterogeneous, each subset was also heterogeneous.

What accounts for the great diversity of antibody molecules made in one animal against DNP, a small well-defined structure? One possibility considered at the time was antigenic heterogeneity: i.e., in the hapten-protein conjugates used to immunize animals each haptenic group, linked to a different residue in the carrier protein, was surrounded by a distinctive set of amino acids and formed a distinct epitope, each eliciting a somewhat different antibody. This possibility was ruled out, at least for the response to the DNP group, by the results shown in Fig. 2: the anti-DNP antibodies elicited against DNP_1-ribonuclease, in which the single DNP group per RNase molecule attached to a particular lysine residue (lysine 41) was just as heterogeneous in affinity for ε-DNP lysine as the antibodies elicited against conventional DNP-protein conjugate having, say, 50–60 DNP groups per protein molecule attached to diverse lysine residues (4).

According to another possibility, antibody molecules fold up imprecisely or sloppily, an idea then favored by immunologists who then still clung to the antigen-template hypothesis (5, 6). The alternative view was that the anti-DNP antibodies in serum were a mixture of many different sets of homogeneous antibodies (monoclonal antibodies in today's parlance), each made by a particular B cell clone (7). Though not required by the clonal selection theory, it was generally assumed by those supporting it that the antibody molecules made by each B cell (or B cell clone) were uniformly folded and would bind the ligand with a single binding constant.

Myeloma proteins provided a way to test the clonal alternative. If this hypothesis were correct, the antibody molecules produced by a single clone of

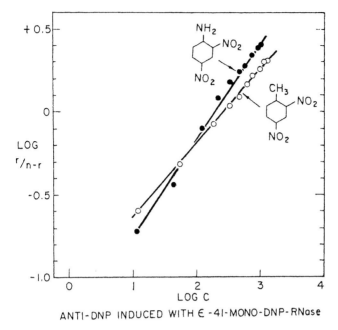

ANTI-DNP INDUCED WITH ∈ -41-MONO-DNP-RNase

Fig. 2. A homogeneous antigen can elicit heterogeneous antibodies. The antigen was bovine pancreatic Rnase having a single DNP group per protein molecule attached to a particular lyineresidue (lyine 41). The anti-DNP antibodies elicited by this antigen were just as heterogeneous with respect to the equilibrium constant for binding ε-DNP lysine as those shown in Fig 1, which were elicited with a DNP protein conjugate having 50-60 DNP groups per protein molecule. From ref. 4

antibody-producing cells should bind the antigen with uniform affinity. The only candidates available at the time for such a test were myeloma proteins. Secreted by myeloma (plasma cell) tumors, these proteins had the same heavy and light chain structure as antibody molecules, but from their electrophoretic behavior and other properties the protein made by each tumor seemed homogeneous and distinctive (8). But, did they have authentic antigen-binding sites? They were regarded by many, even Rod Porter, the astute discoverer of the multichain structure of immunoglobulins (Ig), as abnormal "paraproteins" because they were made by abnormal (cancer) cells. Given the enormous number of different antigens in the biosphere and the prevailing idea that each antibody recognizes a single epitope, or a few structurally similar ones, the chances of finding a myeloma protein that specifically bound any particular epitope – if the protein indeed had an antibody-like binding site – was expected to be extremely small. We nevertheless undertook the search because an attractive means could be visualized for rapidly screening serum samples from patients with myeloma tumors.

A Rapid Screen to Detect Antigen-Binding Sites on Myeloma Proteins

DNP-amino acids undergo a prominent "red" spectral shift when bound to anti-DNP antibodies, probably because of charge-transfer complexes formed by the bound ligand with a tryptophan residue that may be in, or very close to, the antibody binding site (3). The shift appeared to be a distinctive general marker for anti-DNP antibody binding sites since we had consistently seen it with anti-DNP antibodies from diverse sources (produced in immunized rabbits, guinea pigs, chickens, etc.). When, however, serum albumin, the abundant serum protein that binds (weakly) a great many different ligands, binds a DNP-amino acid, the bound ligand's absorption spectrum shifts in the opposite direction (to the "blue"). Thus, it seemed that simple spectrophotometric readings made after addition of ε-DNP-lysine to serum samples from patients having a myeloma tumor would quickly reveal whether this ligand was bound to a myeloma protein that behaved like an antibody (9).

The opportunity to test this screening procedure was facilitated by access to a double-beam Cary spectrophotometer. With the aid of that instrument and specially constructed cuvettes it was possible to test a serum sample in a few minutes. Effective screening required a large number of serum samples and fortunately these were provided by Kurt Osterland, who had for years been collecting them from patients with myeloma tumors. When the screening got underway, it was anticipated, as noted above, that we would be lucky to find one sample out of perhaps a thousand with the desired properties. Instead, one turned up in fewer than the first twenty tested. The active serum, called BRY (after the patient's family name) came from a patient who had left the hospital and was gone without a trace. Only three ml of her serum was available in Osterland's collection. That was sufficient to isolate enough of the myeloma protein (an IgG1 molecule) to show that it had two binding sites per molecule, one in each Fab fragment, and that ε-DNP lysine bound to it in the same way as to conventional anti-DNP antibodies (9). It differed however in the one important feature of particular interest: the equilibrium constant that characterized its binding of ε-DNP lysine was clearly homogeneous (Fig. 3), unlike the heterogeneity that characterized each of the innumerable samples of anti-DNP antibodies isolated from immunized animals. The results supported other mounting evidence for the "one cell-one antibody" rule, the keystone of the clonal selection hypothesis.

The Frequency of Ligand-Binding Myeloma Proteins

The amount of the BRY protein was too limited for structural analyses. To look for additional DNP-binding myeloma proteins, mouse myeloma tumors were more promising than their human counterparts. A large number of these mouse tumors had been accumulated by Michael Potter at the US National Institutes of Health. Each tumor could be propagated indefinitely by transplanting it serially in BALB/c mice, suggesting that virtually unlimited amounts of any myeloma protein having interesting ligand-binding activity could be obtained.

Out of the approximately first 100 mouse myeloma sera screened, two with substantial ε-DNP-lysine-binding activity were identified. The first one found, MOPC-315, bound ε-DNP lysine particularly well, as strongly, indeed, as some anti-DNP antibodies raised in rabbits by conventional immunization procedures (10). The finding of several myeloma proteins with considerable affinity for nitrophenyl groups among the small number of myeloma sera screened was (and is) unexpected because of the general view that i) the total pool of antibodies made by each of us can recognize an enormous number of different antigens and haptens, and ii) the reactivity of each antibody was restricted to one antigen (and a few similar ones). The alternative possibility was that some antibodies can bind to a substantial number of different antigenic groups (epitopes). To examine the latter possibility, we chose, more-or-less at random, a large number of organic molecules (the aim was 57, the number appearing in a then popular advertisement for the Heinz food company) to determine if any of them could competitively inhibit the binding of a radiolabeled DNP ligand to MOPC-315. Several competitors were found by Maria Michaelides, the most active being menadione or vitamine K3 (2-methy-1,4-naphthaquinone) (11). It turned out that this ligand was also bound by conventional antibodies to various nitrophenyl-protein conjugates: 2,4-dinitrophenyl-, 2,6-dinitrophenyl-, and 2,4,6-trinitrophenyl-protein antigens (Fig. 3). These strange cross-reactions indicated a much less precise fit of antigen or hapten to the antibody binding site than is conjured up by the classical lock-in-key metaphor. The imprecision probably corresponds to what was later termed "molecular mimicry" (12). Other examples of such "strange" cross reactions by antibodies, usually encountered serendipitously, have been described. But with the advent of Milstein's and Kohler's powerful procedure for generating monoclonal antibodies, the extent to which individual myeloma proteins and conventional antibodies react with many disparate epitopes ceased to be of much interest. Whether individual antibody-producing cells, B cells, can react with diverse antigens is an issue we shall revisit later.

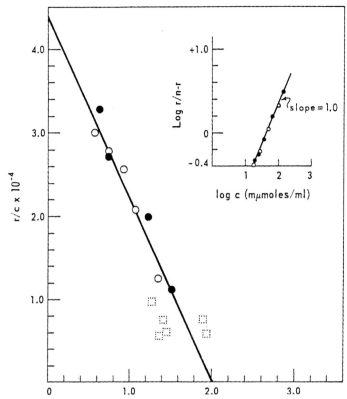

Fig. 3. Homogeneous binding of ε-DNP lysine to a myeloma protein. Data points in closed circles were obtained by fluorescence quenching (as in Figs. 1, 2), those in open circles by equilibrium dialysis. The data are plotted according to the Scatchard equation and replotted in the insert according to the logarithmic form of the Sips distribution. From ref. 9

Antigen-recognition by T cells

In the 1930's, Landsteiner became interested in delayed type hypersensitivity (DTH) skin reactions. Following his pattern of using simple, well-defined chemicals to analyze complex biological responses, he made extensive use of mono-, di, and tri-nitrobenzenes to examine the specificity of these reactions in guinea pigs (13). Animals sensitized with one sensitizer were tested by painting small areas of their skin with that sensitizer and several structurally related compounds, looking 24–48 hrs later for the characteristic skin redness and swelling that marked a positive DTH response. Some of the nitrobenzenes, such as picryl chloride, were notorious as "sensitizers" that caused allergic

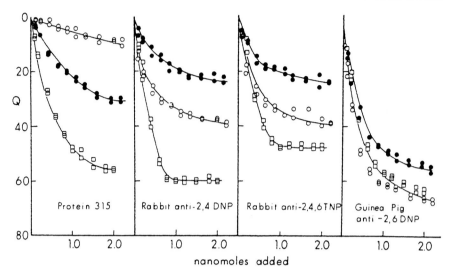

Fig. 4. Anti-DNP binding sites on a myeloma protein (MOPC-315) and on some conventional rabbit and guinea pig antibodies raised against various polynitrophenyl-protein conjugates can also bind vitamin K3 (menadione), a naphthaquinone. From ref. 11

contact dermatitis in workers engaged in their production. The basis for these reactions in humans and guinea pigs was then totally obscure. William Tillett, Chairman of the Department of Medicine at the New York University College of Medicine, once asked at a symposium in New York City in the late 1940's whether these responses were really immune reactions, i.e, manifestations of the same system of which antibodies were the hallmark. The question was entirely reasonable and stemmed from the many failed efforts to transfer DTH reactivity with serum from sensitized to naïve animals. Nevertheless, my answer to the question – yes, they were immune responses – reflected the sentiments of most immunologists at the time who were impressed by the fact that, like antibody responses, the DTH reactions were characterized by specificity and "memory". Figure 5 illustrates their specificity: I had been sensitized by 2,4-dinitrofluorobenzene while synthesizing this compound (before it became available commercially) and, as shown in the Figure, I responded positively to patch tests of my own skin with various nitrobenzenes only if they were able to form 2,4-dinitrophenyl derivatives of (skin) proteins (14) but not if the derivatives were 2,6-dinitrophenyl or 2,4,6-trinitrophenyl (Fig. 5) (15). (Various cross-sensitivity reaction among these closely related molecules can be found, however, in other individuals.) The evidence for memory was simply the more rapid induction of DTH on encountering a particular sensitizer again, long after initially encountering it.

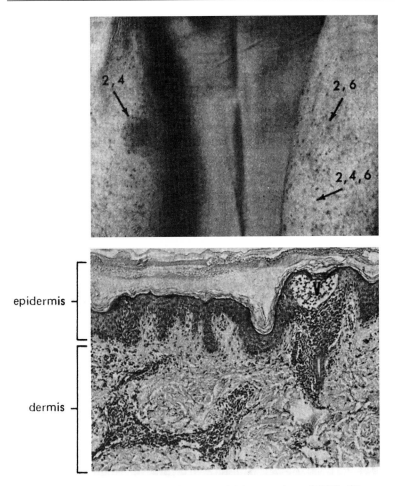

Fig. 5. Specificity in delayed type hypersensitivity reactions (DTH). (Upper panel) The subject had been sensitized previously with 2,4-dinitrofluorobenzene. Subsequently, a positive reaction was elicited by 2,4-dinitrochlorobenzene, but not by 2,6-dinitrochlorobenzene or 2,4,6-trinitrochlorobenzene. Each of these compounds reacts similarly with amino groups of lysine residues. (Lower panel) Biopsy of the positive skin reaction showing the characteristic lesion of allergic contact dermatitis. From ref. X

A significant step in establishing the distinction between B and T cells was the finding that T cells but not B cells, could transfer DTH to a particular antigen from sensitized donor to naïve recipients, suggesting that T cells expressed antigen-specific receptors (T cell receptors or TCR). The development of procedures for generating mouse T cell clones and expanding them in culture with retention of normal function opened opportunities to study antigen recognition by isolated cells ex vivo. Our lab concentrated on CD8 T cells, and for several years new postdoctoral fellows coming to the lab were encouraged to generate murine T cell clones. Many were produced and some grew especially well and could be maintained in culture for years.

One of the better clones was called 2C. Generated initially by Mischa Sitkovsky, then a recent immigrant from the Soviet Union, it was nurtured and developed by David Kranz, who also generated a monoclonal antibody that reacted exclusively with the TCR on 2C cells (16). These cells served as the basis for a collaborative effort with Susumu Tonegawa's lab that resulted in cloning the genes for the α and β subunits of the clone's TCR, called the 2C TCR. Later, transgenic mice expressing the 2C αβ TCR were produced in Dennis Loh's lab at Washington University Medical School in St. Louis (17), and from these mice additional clones and cell lines expressing this receptor were generated in our lab.

Antigen Recognition by a T Cell Clone

What does the 2C TCR recognize? Following Zinkernagel's and Doherty's finding that MHC proteins "restrict" antigen recognition by T cells, and the findings by Unanue and Townsend and others that short peptides arising as proteolytic fragments from proteins, intracellular or other, associate with proteins encoded in the major histocompatibility complex (MHC proteins), it has become evident that TCR generally recognize peptide-MHC complexes. In these complexes, both the peptide and adjoining areas of the MHC protein's binding site constitute, together, the epitope that is recognized. When the 2C clone was first derived, it was readily apparent that its TCR recognized L^d, a non-self (or allogeneic) class I MHC protein present on the cells used to immunize mice that lacked L^d (16). But identification of the peptide associated with L^d required the heroic efforts of Keiko Udaka and Ted Tsomides, who systematically analyzed the myriad of peptides in mouse spleen extracts, separating them chromatographically (by HPLC) and identifying active fractions by the cytolytic responses of 2C cells. From spleens of around 1000 mice they ultimately purified two peptides. Their overlapping amino acid sequences led to the identity of their source, which turned out to a mitochondrial "housekeeping" protein (α-ketoglutarate dehydrogenase), expressed in all cells (18, 19).

As with all αβ TCR, the 2C TCR has to recognize an indigenous (self) MHC protein in order to complete its maturation in the thymus. For T cells expressing the 2C TCR this self MHC was shown in breeding experiments with 2C transgenic mice to be K^b (20). This TCR can thus recognize peptide-K^b as well as peptide-L^d complexes, including at least one peptide (from α-ketoglutarate dehydrogenase) that associates with L^d and K^b. Some years later, Tallquist et al identified another peptide, from a different mitochondrial protein, that is recognized by the 2C TCR in association with K^{bm3} and also with K^b (21).

Degeneracy in Antigen Recognition by 2C T Cells

How many other peptide-MHC complexes do 2C cells recognize? The recognition of complexes by a TCR is easily evaluated from the cytolytic responses of CD8 T cells to "target" cells that express an appropriate MHC protein and are incubated with various synthetic peptides. By binding to the MHC on the target cell surface, the peptides form peptide-MHC complexes on the target cells: if the complexes are recognized by cytolytic T cells the target cells are destroyed. Simple cytolytic assays of this kind have determined that the 2C TCR can recognize a great many different peptide-MHC complexes involving at least 12 peptides (some with overlapping sequences) in association with three MHC proteins (K^b, L^d, and K^{bm3}) (22, 23, and Fig. 6). They also respond to still another MHC protein, from another MHC locus (H-2^r) (Eisen & Cornell, unpublished observations), probably in association with still other peptides. Furthermore, it also appears from the maturation of these cells in mice lacking classical class I MHC proteins that they can recognize an as yet unidentified class I MHC of the so-called nonclassical type, which possibly binds some glycolipids instead of short peptides in its binding groove (24). The ability to recognize and respond to so many different structures deserves to be called "degeneracy." Degeneracy has been seen previously to various extents, as in reactions attributed to "molecular mimicry" (12) and in Wucherpfennig and Strominger's elegant study with T cells that react with a peptide from myelin basic protein as well as many viral peptides (25). A recent paper by Joshi et al demonstrates quite strikingly that individual CD4 T cell clones can be stimulated to proliferate by peptides of widely divergent sequences (26). There is no good reason to doubt that many TCR would exhibit similar degrees of degeneracy if examined thoroughly.

T Cells Can Discriminate Sharply Between Similar Structures

Although 2C T cells exhibit much degeneracy, they can also display exquisite specificity in discriminating between very similar structures. For example, these T cells lyse target cells presenting a peptide-MHC complex, call it A, but not the same target cells that present the same number of a slightly different

A Partial List of Peptide-MHC Complexes
Eliciting Responses from 2CT Cells

MHC	Peptides	
	Name	Sequence
K^b	p2Ca *	LSPFPFDL
	dEV8**	EQYKFYSV
	• SYRGL*	SIYRYYGL
K^bm3	dEV8	EQYKFYSV
Ld	p2Cb	VAITRIEQLSPFPFDL
	RL12	RIEQLSPFPFDL
	QL9	QLSPFPFDL
	p2Ca	LSPFPFDL
	SL7	SPFPFDL
	PL4	PFDL
	p2Ca-Y4	LSPYPFDL
	• QL9-Y5	QLSPYPFDL
	• I₁-QL9-Y5	QLSPY(I₁)PFDL
H-2r	?	?
Nonclassical MHC-I	?	?

Except for peptides marked by • all peptides listed have been isolated from murine cells or tissue or cleaved from p2Cb by 20S proteasomes (see text from Kageyama et al., submitted).

Fig. 6. See Table

complex, call it A', where the difference between A and A' is a single O atom resulting from a phenylalanine-tyrosine substitution in the peptide (22, Fig. 7). This difference equals the highest degree of specificity seen in the most discriminating reactions of antibodies or enzymes.

ANTIGEN-SPECIFIC T-CELL RECEPTORS

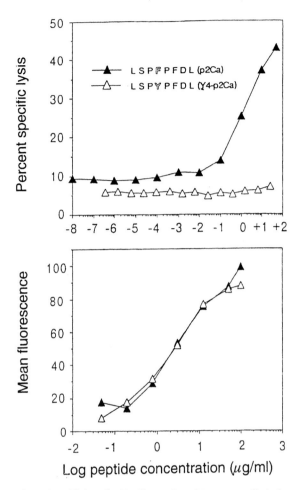

Fig. 7. Specificity of a T cell reaction. (Upper panel) A clone of cytotoxic CD8+ T cells (2C) lyse target cells that present the octapeptide p2Ca in association with Kb (class I MHC) (closed triangles), but not the same target cells that present the octapeptide Y4-p2Ca in association with the same class I MHC. The octapeptides differ by the tyrosine/phenlyalanine substitution shown, or by 1 O atom. (Lower panel) The p2Ca and Y4-p2Ca peptides bind equally well to Kb on the target cells. From ref.22 (see also ref. 23)

Specificity Versus Degeneracy

How can the same TCR display exquisite specificity in some reactions and extensive degeneracy in others? An explanation for specificity is not hard to discern. Specificity, the capacity to discriminate between two similar structures, depends not only on the difference in strength (call it affinity) of the two reactions but on how the reactions are detected. Since all detection systems have a threshold, below which reactions cannot be detected, a pair of ligands whose strengths of reaction straddle the threshold can be sharply distinguished. This, in fact, is the situation with the above cited example of the A and A' epitopes that differ only by a phenylalanine-tyrosine substitution (i.e., by 1 O atom): the 2C TCR has the lowest measureable affinity for the epitope (A) that elicited target cell lysis (an equilibrium constant of about 3×10^{-3} M^{-1}) (27), and probably an immeasurably lower affinity for the epitope (A') that failed to elicit target cell lysis.

Degeneracy is more intriguing because of its implications for the hypothesis that has served as the guiding paradigm for immunology over the past 40 years. The degenerate and specific reactions we are referring to here have been detected primarily by cytolytic assays. The extent of target cell destruction in these assays depends not only upon their displaying a peptide-MHC complex (epitope) that is recognized by the TCR, but upon the number of copies of the epitope per target cell ("epitope density"). It also depends upon the affinity of the TCR for the epitope (i.e., on the equilibrium constant for the TCR-epitope reaction). And from studies carried out with Yuri Sykulev, Richard Cohen, and Ted Tsomides (28) it appears that high epitope densities are required for low-affinity reactions while low epitope densities suffice for high-affinity reactions (29). This inverse relationship calls to mind the law of mass action, the fundamental rule for reversible chemical reactions involving molecules and ions that are freely diffusible in solution. Its application to reactions between the TCR and peptide-MHC complexes, each embedded as an integral membrane protein in the surface of a T cell and an antigen-presenting cell (APC), respectively, is not to be undertaken lightly (30). Nevertheless, this rule, with some simplifying assumptions, seems to provide a useful framework for viewing T cell reactions with APC (29)(Fig. 8).

One Cell-Many Specificities

The central principle of the clonal selection hypothesis, the "1 cell-1 antibody" rule, has been repeatedly confirmed. It has been extended, almost subliminally, to mean "1 cell-1 specificity", because an antibody molecule characteristically

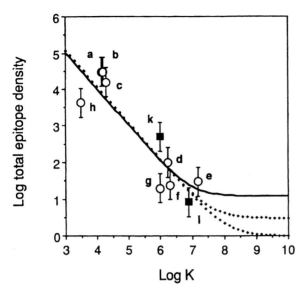

Fig. 8. An inverse relationship between the equilibrium constant (K) for the TCR-peptide/MHC interaction and the number of copies of the cognate peptide-MHC complex required on target cells (epitope density) for half-maximal lysis of the target cells in a standard cytolytic assay. From ref. 29

reacts, as ordinarily measured, with a single antigen and a few structurally similar ones. For T cells, the corresponding 1 cell-1 TCR rule is also correct (although some T cells can have two TCR owing to the absence of allelic exclusion for the α subunit of $\alpha\beta$ TCR). However, the responsiveness of T cells to diverse epitopes indicates that the "1 cell-1 specificity" rule for these cells is far from correct. A more reasonable phrase would be "1 cell-many specificities", with the magnitude of "many" still to be determined.

Why T Cells Exhibit More Degeneracy Than Antibodies

Given the great structural similarity between antibodies and TCR, why should T cells, via their TCR, display so much more degeneracy than antibodies? The likely answer (aside from the arguable possibility that TCR binding-sites are more flexible and conformationally adaptable to bound ligands than are antibody binding sites) is that very few of the many TCR molecules on a T cell's surface (probably fewer than 10 out of around 100,000) have to be initially engaged in a stable TCR-epitope complex to trigger a detectable T cell response

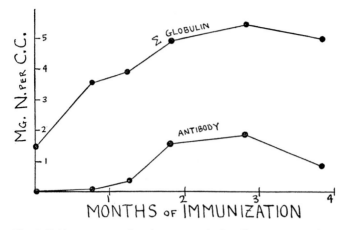

Fig. 9. Evidence suggesting degeneracy in B cell responses to immunization. The serum antibodies produced by rabbits immunized with ovalbumin account for less than half the increase in serum globulin resulting from injection of antigen. From ref. 33

(31). This great sensitivity stems from powerful amplification effects of cellular signal transduction cascades. Moreover, the capacity to recognize – i.e., to respond to – so many different epitopes reflects the importance of epitope density on antigen presenting cells. At a sufficiently high epitope density a very weakly bound epitope can probably form a sufficient number of stable TCR-epitope engagements to trigger some T cell responses (32).

Are B Cells Similarly Degenerate?

The foregoing view may also apply to B cells. An indication that they can exhibit degeneracy can be seen in the levels of serum proteins following injections of antigens in conventional immunization procedures. It has been observed that, following injections of antigen, total globulin levels in antisera can greatly exceed levels of the antibodies that react specifically with the administered antigen (33) (Fig. 9). It may be that Jerne, in proposing the anti-idiotype network, was influenced by this difference. A more likely explanation than an idiotype/anti-idiotype network is that in vivo B cell responses are substantially degenerate, as are the T cell responses considered above. Thus, administration of an antigen (call it X) results in stimulating not only those B cells whose secreted immunoglobulins (Igs) function as recognizable anti-X antibodies, but probably also many other B cells, whose secreted Igs have too low an affinity for X to qualify as anti-X antibodies. When normal B cell clones become available it may be feasible to test this possibility.

In closing, I want to mention the delightful visit last evening to Schönbrunn Palace. The music was wonderful, but I had some trouble following the words and my mind wandered a bit. The palace brought to mind a fairy tale analogy for T and B cell activation. According to the tale a sleeping beauty, asleep for a hundred years, is finally awakened by the kiss of a handsome prince. In the immune system parallel, the sleeping beauty is a naïve T cell or B cell, the handsome prince is the singular antigen recognized by the cell's antigen-specific receptor, and the kiss is the antigen-receptor interaction. If degeneracy in antigen recognition were to apply to the fairy tale, the sleeping beauty would not have had to wait for a particular handsome prince but might have been awakened by any of several princes, not necessarily handsome and possibly even ugly, and or even by some carpenters or cobblers or others.

Finally, I wish to thank Professors Eibl, Thorbecke, and Mayr for the invitation to participate in this memorable meeting, with its delightful combination of interesting science and stimulating opportunities to see some great art and to hear some wonderful Mozart.

Acknowledgements

The work from my laboratory cited in this article has been supported by research grants from the National Institutes of Health of the US Public Health Service. The article is largely based on ref. 34 and directly incorporates some parts of that reference.

References

1. Landsteiner K (1943) The specificity of serological reactions. Harvard Univ Press Cambridge MA:5
2. Foote J. Eisen HN (2000) Breaking the affinity ceiling for antibodies and T cell receptors. Proc Natl Acad Sci USA 97:10679
3. Eisen HN Siskind GW (1964) Variations in affinities of antibodies during the immune response. Biochem 3:996
4. Eisen HN (1966) The immune response to a simple antigenic determinant. The Harvey Lectures Series 60:1
5. Haurowitz F Breinl F. (1933) Zeit physiol Chem 214:111
6. Pauling L (1940) J Amer Chem Soc 62:2643
7. Burnet FM (1959) The clonal selection theory of aquired immunity. Vanderbilt Univ Press, Nashville

8. Natvig JB Kunkel HG (1973) Human immunoglobulins: classes, subclasses, genetic variants, and idiotypes. Adv Immunol 16:1
9. Eisen HN Little JR, Osterland CK Simms ES (1967) A myeloma protein with antibody activity. Cold Spring Harbor Symp Quant Biol 32:75
10. Eisen HN, Potter P Simms E (1968) Mouse myeloma proteins with anti-hapten antibody activity: the protein produced by plasma cell tumor MOPC-315. Biochemistry 7:4126
11. Michaelides MC Eisen HN (1974) The strange cross-reaction of menadione (Vitmin K3) and 2,4-dinitrophenyl ligands with a myeloma protein and some conventional antibodies. J Exp Med 140:687
12. Fujinami RS, Oldstone MB (1989) Molecular mimicry as a mechanism for viral-induced autoimmunity. Immunol Rev 8:3
13. Chase MW (1985) Immunology and experimental dermatology. Ann Rev Immunol 3:1
14. Eisen HN Orris L, Belman S (1952) Elicitation of delayed allergic skin reactions with haptens: the dependence of elicitation on hapten combination with protein. J Exp Med 95:473
15. Eisen HN (1990) General Immunology. J.B. Lippincott Co. Philadelphia (also published as a section of Microbiology, 4th edition, by Davis, Dulbecco, Eisen, and Ginsberg):210
16. Kranz DM, Sherman DH, Sitkovsky MV, Pasternack MS, Eisen HN (1984) Immunoprecipitation of cell surface structures of cloned cytotoxic T lymphocytes by clone-specific antisera. Proc Natl Acad Sci USA 81:573
17. Sha WC, Nelson CA, Newberry RD, Kranz DM, Russell JH, Loh DY (1988) Selective expression of an antigen receptor on CD8-bearing T lymphocytes in transgenic mice. Nature 335:271
18. Udaka K, Tsomides TJ, Eisen HN (1992) A naturally occurring peptide recognized by alloreactive CD8$^+$ cytotoxic T lymphocytes in association with a class I MHC protein. Cell 69:989
19. Udaka K, Tsomides TJ, Walden P, Fukusen N, Eisen HN (1993) A ubiquitous protein is the source of naturally occurring peptides that are recognized by a CD8 T cell clone. Proc Natl Acad Sci USA 90:11271.
20. Sha WC, Nelson CA, Newberry RD, Pullen JK, Pease LR, Russell JH, Loh DY (1990) Positive selection of transgenic receptor-bearing thymocytes by Kb antigen is altered by Kb mutations that involve peptide binding. Proc Natl Acad Sci USA 87:6186
21. Tallquist MD, Yun TJ, Pease LR (1996) A single T cell receptor recognizes structurally distinct MHC/peptide complexes with high specificity. J Exp Med 184:1017
22. Wu M, Tsomides TJ, Eisen HN (1995) Tissue distribution of natural peptides derived from a ubiquitous dehydrogenase, including a novel liver-specific peptide that demonstrates the pronounced specificity of low affinity T cell reactions. J Immunol 154:4495
23. Eisen HN, Sykulev Y, Tsomides T (1996) Antigen specific T-cell receptors and their reactions with complexes formed by peptides with major histocompatibility complex proteins. Adv Protein Chem 49:1
24. Maurice MM, Gould DS, Carroll J, Vugmeyster Y, Ploegh HL (2000) Positive selection of an MHC class 1-restricted TCR in the absence of classical MHC class 1 molecules. Submitted
25. Wucherpfennig KW, Strominger JL (1995) Molecular mimicry in T cell-mediated auto-immunity: viral peptides activate human T cell clones specific for myelin basic protein. Cell 80:695

26. Joshi SK, Suresh PR, Chauhan VS (2000) Flexibility in MHC and TCR recognition: degenerate specificity at the T cell level in the recognition of promiscuous T H epitopes exhibiting no primary sequence homology. J Immunol in press

27. Sykulev Y, Brunmark A, Jackson M, Cohen RJ, Peterson PA, Eisen HN (1994) Kinetics and affinity of reactions between an antigen-specific T-cell-receptor and peptide-MHC complexes. Immunity 1:15

28. Tsomides TJ, Aldovini A, Johnson RP, Walker BD, Young RA, Eisen HN (1994) Naturally processed viral peptides recognized by cytotoxic T lymphocytes on cells chronically infected by human immunodeficiency virus type 1 (HIV-1). J Exp Med 180:1283

29. Sykulev Y, Cohen RJ, Eisen HN (1995) The law of mass action governs antigen-stimulated cytolytic activity of $CD8^+$ cytotoxic lymphocytes. Proc Natl Acad Sci USA 92:11990

30. Bell GI, Dembo M, Bongrad P (1984) Cell adhesion. Competition between nonspecific repulsion and specific bonding. Biophys J 45:1051

31. Sykulev Y, Joo M, Vturina I, Tsomides T, Eisen HN (1996) Evidence that a single peptide-MHC complex on a target cell can elicit a cytolytic T cell response. Immunity 4:565

32. Cho BK, Lian K-C, Lee P, Brunmark A, McKinley C, Chen J, Kranz DM, Eisen HN. Submitted. Differences in antigen-recognition and cytolytic activity of $CD8^+$ and $CD8^-$ T cells that express the same antigen-specific receptor.

33. Boyd WC, Bernard H (1937) J Immunol 33:111

34. Eisen HN (2001) Specificity and degeneracy in antigen recognition. Ann Rev Immunol 19:1

Induction and Suppression of an Autoimmune Disease by Oligomerized T Cell Epitopes: Enhanced In Vivo Potency of Encephalitogenic Peptides

K. Falk[1], O. Rötzschke[1], L. Santambrogio[2], M.E. Dorf[3], C. Brosnan[4], and J. L. Strominger[1,2]

Abstract

T cell epitope peptides derived from proteolipid protein (PLP130–151) or myelin basic protein (MBP86–100) induce experimental autoimmune encephalomyelitis (EAE) in "susceptible" strains of mice (e.g., SJL/J). In this study, we show that the encephalitogenic effect of these epitopes when injected subcutaneously in complete Freund's adjuvant was significantly enhanced if administered to the animal in a multimerized form as a T cell epitope oligomer (i.e., as multiple repeats of the epitope, such as 16-mers). Oligomer-treated SJL/J mice developed EAE faster and showed a more severe progression of the disease than animals treated with peptide alone. In addition, haplotype-matched B10.S mice, "resistant" to EAE induction by peptide, on injection of 16-mers developed a severe form of EAE. Even more striking, however, was the dramatic suppression of incidence and severity of the disease, seen after single intravenous injections of only 50 µg of the PLP139-151 16-mer, administered to SJL/J mice 7 d after the induction of the disease. Although relapse occurred at about day 45, an additional injection several days before that maintained the suppression. Importantly, the specific suppressive effect of oligomer treatment was also evident if EAE was induced with spinal cord homogenate instead of

[1] Department of Molecular and Cellular Biology, Harvard University, Cambridge, Massachusetts 02138

[2] Department of Cancer Immunology and AIDS, Dana-Farber Cancer Institute, Boston, Massachusetts 02115

[3] Department of Pathology, Harvard Medical School, Boston, Massachusetts 02115

[4] Department of Pathology, Albert Einstein College of Medicine, Bronx, New York 10461
Address correspondence to Jack L. Strominger, Department of Molecular and Cellular Biology, Harvard University, 7 Divinity Ave., Cambridge, MA 02138. Phone: 617–495-2733; Fax: 617-496-8351; E-mail: jlstrom@fas.harvard.edu

the single peptide antigen. By contrast, the PLP139–151 peptide accelerated rather than retarded the progression of disease.

Key words: apoptosis · anergy · high zone tolerance · experimental autoimmune encephalomyelitis · multimer

Introduction

T cell epitope oligomers are linear polypeptide chains, which consist of multiple copies of a T cell epitope. They contain up to 32 repeats of the epitope connected to each other by a flexible spacer sequence (sp)[1] of ~ 13 amino acids. Previously, oligomers (16-mers) of an epitope derived from the influenza virus hemagglutinin protein (HA306–318) have been shown to induce an exceptionally strong CD4[+] T cell proliferative response in vitro (at almost 1,000-fold lower concentration than the peptide) (1). To evaluate whether oligomers can also act as stronger immunogens in vivo, experimental animals models were needed.

Experimental autoimmune encephalitis (EAE) is the best studied experimental animal model of a T cell-mediated autoimmune disease. It serves as the animal model of human multiple sclerosis (2) and can be initiated by a subcutaneous injection of encephalitogenic peptides. In most cases, these peptides are "self-antigens" derived from myelin proteins (3), such as proteolipid protein (PLP [4, 5]), myelin basic protein (MBP [6, 7]), or myelin oligodendrocyte protein (MOG [8]). These peptides, when associated to MHC class II molecules, are the target structure for autoreactive CD4[+] T cells.

The extent of the pathological changes after the induction of the disease can be evaluated by scoring the clinical symptoms typical for EAE. This clinical score reflects the "encephalitogenicity" of the antigen and can be used to estimate its in vivo potency. However, not all mouse strains respond equally to a given encephalitogenic peptide antigen. Incidence rate and severity of the disease are strongly affected by the genotype of the recipient mouse. Primarily, the H2 haplotype dictates whether the strain is "permissive" or "nonpermissive" for disease induction by the particular antigen, but in addition other genetic factors play a role ultimately determining whether a permissive strain is actually also "susceptible" (9). The secondary mechanisms underlying "sus-

---

[1] Abbreviations used in this paper: EAE, experimental autoimmune encephalomyelitis; HA, influenza hemagglutinin protein; LNC, lymph node cell; MBP, myelin basic protein; MOG, myelin oligodendrocyte protein; PLP, proteolipid protein; sp, spacer sequence.

ceptibility" and "resistance" are not known at the present time, but they appear to affect the overall sensitivity for the induction of an immune response. As a consequence, the induction of EAE in resistant strains, such as B10.S, requires the coinjection of proinflammatory cytokines such as IL-12 (10) or might require exceptionally strong immunogens.

The use of the EAE system for the evaluation of the in vivo potency also allows testing the potential of an antigen to suppress the immune response. In addition to therapeutic approaches using broadly immunosuppressing mechanisms such as the administration of antiinflammatory cytokines (11) or the neutralization of proinflammatory cytokines (12), other more targeted approaches were introduced to "silence" specifically the autoreactive T cells. Most of these approaches aim at the induction of "high zone tolerance" (13), i.e., the induction of anergy (14) or the apoptotic elimination (15) of T cells by overstimulation after exposure to high concentrations of antigen. To achieve tolerance, the antigens have to be administered either by oral uptake (16–18), by intranasal deposition (19), or by intravenous or subcutaneous injection (14, 15, 20, 21). Using these routes of administration, several antigens have already been used successfully in the EAE system to induce tolerance. The list includes peptides (14, 15, 20) or peptide derivates modified by acylation (22) or amino acid substitution (23), but also proteins (21, 24) and protein-protein (25) and immunoglobulin–protein chimeras (26). However, these experiments were usually carried out in transgenic animals, which express only the TCR specific for the peptide antigen (15, 20). Few reports exist in which "normal" nontransgenic mice were treated successfully with encephalitogenic self-peptides after the disease was already induced (27). In these cases, however, a relatively high internal level of the antigen had to be maintained by the frequent administration of high doses of the peptide.

In this study, we tested the efficiency of multimerized forms of the encephalitogenic T cell epitopes PLP139–151 (4) and MBP86–100 (7) on both the induction and suppression of EAE. The disease induction was tested with several mouse strains, including resistant B10.S mice in which the peptides were known to have no encephalitogenic effect. The effect on the suppression of the autoimmune disease was tested with normal SJL/J mice, not biased by the transgenic expression of a particular TCR.

Materials and Methods

Antigens. For stability reasons, the residue Cys140 in the PLP139–151 epitope was substituted by Ser (a substitution that has no or little effect on the encephalitogenicity of the epitope [4]). The synthetic peptides PLP139–151 (C140S)

(HSLGKWLGHPDKF), PLP139–151 (HCLGKWLGHPDKF), sp-PLP139–151 (C140S)-sp (GGGPGGHSLGKWLGHPDKFGGPGGG), PLP178–191 (C183S) (NTWTTSQSIAFPSK), MBP86–100 (NPVVHFFKNIVTPRT), and MBP86–101 (NPVVHFFKNIVTPRTP) were produced by using standard solid phase F-moc chemistry and purchased from the Biopolymers Laboratory at the Harvard Medical School. All peptides were purified on a C_4-HPLC column (Vydac).

Oligomerized T cell epitopes were produced in *Escherichia coli* bacteria using recombinant techniques as described previously (1). In brief, double-stranded oligonucleotide units encoding the T cell epitopes of the PLP139–151 (C140S) oligomers and MBP86–100 oligomers were generated by annealing two complementary strands of synthetic oligonucleotides (PLP139–151 (C140S), + strand: 5'-TCACTCTCTGGGTAAATGGCTGGGGTCACCCGGATAAATTCGG, and – strand: 5'-GAATTTATCCGGGTGACCCAGCCATTTACCCAGAGAGTGA-CC; MBP86–100, + strand: 5'-CAACCCGGTTGTTCACTTCTTCAAAAACAT-CGTAACTCCGCGTACTGG, and – strand: 5'-AGTACGCGGAGTTACGATGTTT-TTGAAGAAGTGAACAAGCGGGTTGCC). They were linked to the NH_2-terminal side of a spacer sequence (amino acid sequence of the S3 spacer: GGPGGGPGGGPGG) by cloning the oligonucleotide into the BsrDI site of a modified pCITE vector (Novagen), which contained the DNA encoding the S3 spacer (the construction of full-length oligomeric DNA is described in reference 1). The same spacer was also used in MBP86–101 oligomers, which were provided by Dr. Shan Chung (Peptimmune, Inc., Cambridge, MA). The proteins were produced in TOP10 (pLysS) bacteria (Invitrogen) by using a pET22b expression vector (Novagen). The purification of the expressed protein was carried out using Ni^{2+}-NTA-agarose (Quiagen) by using a His tag located at the COOH terminus of the constructs. Endotoxin and other impurities were removed from the polypeptide oligomers by separation on a reversed-phase C_4-HPLC column (Vydac).

Spinal cords from mice were isolated, homogenized, and lyophilized as described elsewhere (28).

T Cell Lines and Clones. The T cell lines SP/2, SP/3, PLP/a, and PLP/c were generated and maintained as described previously (29). In brief, SJL mice were immunized subcutaneously with PLP139–151 (C140S) peptide emulsified in CFA. Lymph node cells (LNCs) were isolated on day 8–12 after immunization and initially stimulated with 50 µg/ml PLP139–151 (C140S) in the presence of 0.8–1.0 % autologous mouse serum. The cultures were subsequently restimulated after 6 d and then every 2–3 wk with 10 µg/ml PLP139–151 (C140S) and irradiated syngeneic splenocytes (1,200 rad). They were expanded in DMEM (supplemented with 20mM glutamine, 1 mM sodium pyruvate, 0.1 mM nonessential amino acids, 10 mM Hepes buffer, 10 % (FCS [Sigma Chemical Co.]) plus

5–10 % of a supernatant derived from concanavalin A-activated mouse spleno-cytes. The T cell line SP/178 was generated in the same way except that PLP178-191 was used instead of PLP139–151 (C140S). The T cell clones SP2.2A8 and 8A1 were obtained by limiting dilution of T cell lines specific for the PLP139–151 antigen at a density of 0.5 cells/well and maintained as described for the T cell line. T cell hybridomas hPLP/1, hPLP/a9.4, and hPLP/c4 were generated by a polyethylene glycol fusion of the T cell lines PLP/a and PLP/c, respectively, with TCR-α/β^- BW1100 thymoma cells, selected in the presence of histone acetyltransferase (HAT) and cloned by limiting dilution as described previously (29).

Mice. SJL/J, PL/J, SWR, B10.S, B10, BALB/c, A.SW, and AKR/J mice (6–8 wk of age) were purchased from The Jackson Laboratory and housed in the animal facility at Harvard University or at Harvard Medical School. They were main-tained in accordance with the Guidelines of the Committees on Animals of Harvard University, and the Committee on Care and Use of Laboratory Animal Resources, National Research Council (Department of Health and Human Services Publication 85–23, revised 1987).

In Vitro Assays. T cell proliferation assays were performed in 96-well round-bottomed plates using 5×10^5 irradiated (1,200 rad) splenocytes and 5×10^4 T cells per well in DMEM/10 % FCS. After 48 h, 5 μCi [^{3}H]thymidine was added per well and the assay was harvested after 72 h and counted in a microbetaplate reader (Wallac). The in vitro proliferation assays of primary LNC cultures were performed in the same way except that 5×10^5 nonirradiated LNCs were plated per well, [^{3}H]thymidine was added after 72 h, and the assay was harvested after 96 h. The response of T cell hybridomas (5×10^5 cells/well) was tested with 5×10^5 splenocytes as target cells by collecting 30 μl of supernatant after 24 h for the determination of IL-2 release in a proliferation assay with CTLL.

Induction of EAE. Mice were injected in the base of the tail and the nape of the neck with indicated amounts of peptide, T cell epitope oligomer, or spinal cord homogenate together with 400 μg *Mycobacterium tuberculosis* H37Ra (Difco Laboratories) in an emulsion consisting of equal parts of PBS and CFA (Sigma Chemical Co.). Each mouse was also injected intravenously with 200 ng of *Pertussis* toxin (List Biological Laboratories) on day 1 or on days 1 and 3 after immunization. Mice were observed once or twice a day for clinical signs of EAE and scored on a scale of 1–5 according to the severity of the clinical signs as described previously (28).

Suppression of EAE by Intravenous Injections. EAE was induced in SJL/J mice by the subcutaneous application of peptide antigens or homogenized mouse spinal cord emulsified in CFA followed by the injection of *Pertussis* toxin as described above. For the intravenous administration, the antigens were dissolved in PBS at a concentration of 0.5–1.0 mg/ml and injected into the tail vein at the dosage and time (day) indicated in the text.

Cytokine Detection. Samples of the supernatant from primary LNC cultures described above were taken after 96 h. The amount of released IL-4 and IFN-γ was determined in a sandwich ELISA using pairs of specific capture and biotinylated detection antibodies (PharMingen) and streptavidin–horseradish peroxidase (Sigma Chemical Co.). The ELISA was developed with TMB (Kirkegaard & Perry Laboratories) and measured at 450 nm using an MRX ELISA reader (Dynatech). IL-2, released by T cell hybridomas, was determined by collecting 30-μl samples of the supernatant 24 h after commencement of the T cell assay by testing the samples in a secondary proliferation assay with IL-2-dependent CTLL cells. Recombinant mIL-2 (Genzyme) was used as reference.

Immunohistochemistry. For assessment of inflammation, the brain and spinal cord were fixed in formalin, embedded in paraffin, and 7-μm sections were stained with hematoxylin and eosin according to standard pathological procedures. For assessment of demyelination, animals were perfused under anesthesia through the ascending aorta with 40 ml of Trump's fixative (4 % paraformaldehyde, 1 % glutaraldehyde in 0.1 M phosphate buffer, pH 7.4). Slices of the brain and spinal cord were postfixed in cold 1 % osmium tetroxide for 1 h, dehydrated through a graded series of ethyl alcohol, and embedded in epoxy resin. 1-μm sections were stained with toluidine blue and examined by light microscopy in a blinded fashion.

Results

Proliferative Response of PLP139–151-specific T Cells In Vitro. In a series of proliferation assays, the biological activity of a PLP139–151(C140S) 16-mer was tested with several different T cell lines and clones (generated as described in Materials and Methods; Fig. 1 A). Compared with the peptide, all T cell lines specific for the PLP139–151 epitope responded better (lines SP/2, SP/3), or at least equally well, to the stimulation with the oligomer (lines PLP/a, PLP/c). No proliferation was induced by the PLP139–151(C140S) 16-mer in the control line, SP/178, which is specific for PLP178–191. As had been established previously

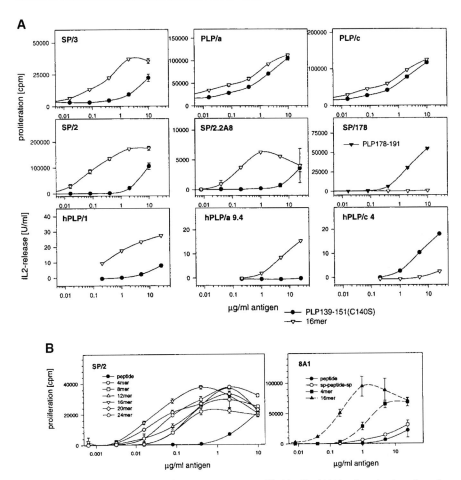

Fig. 1. In vitro experiments with PLP139–151-specific T cells. (A) T cells raised against the PLP139–151(C140S) peptide were challenged with titrated amounts of the PLP139–151(C140S) peptide or the PLP139–151(C140S) 16-mer. The specific response of the T cell lines SP/3, PLP/a, PLP/c, and SP/2, and of the T cell clone SP/2.2A8 was measured in a proliferation assay. The response of the T cell hybridomas hPLP/1, hPLP/a9.4, and hPLP/c4 was determined by their IL-2 release. Also shown is the proliferative response of the line SP/178, specific for PLP178–191. SJL/J splenocytes were used as target cells. (B) Dose-response of PLP139–151-specific T cells to oligomers with an increasing number of repetitive epitope units. SP/2 T cells (left) were tested as described above with the PLP139–151(C140S) peptide and a set of PLP139–151(C140S) oligomers. The right panel shows the proliferative response of the clone 8A1. In addition to the PLP139–151(C140S) peptide, the 4-mer, and the 16-mer, this clone was also tested with a PLP139–151(C140S) peptide containing the NH_2– and COOH-terminal extensions of the spacer sequence (sp-peptide-sp: GGG-PGG-PLP139–151[C140S]-GGPGGG).

for another apitope (HA306–318; reference 1), the gain in sensitivity detected for some of these lines was significant. The T cell line SP2, for example, required ~100-fold lower concentrations of the 16-mer to induce a proliferation equivalent to that of the peptide. A more detailed picture of the proliferative response to the PLP139–152(C140S) 16-mer and peptide was obtained by analyzing single T cell clones. In particular, the response of low-avidity T cell clones improved to the 16-mer. As shown, some of these clones recognized 100-fold less 16-mer than peptide similar to the SP/2 line (SP2/2A8, hPLP/1), and for some clones (e.g., hPLP/a9.4) the specificity for 16-mer appeared even almost absolute. In contrast, other T cell clones (e.g., hPLP/c4) failed to efficiently recognize the 16-mer. For those clones, however, the failure to respond to the oligomer was found to be due to the extension of the actual T cell epitope by the spacer sequence, which presumably caused steric hindrance of the TCR-MHC-antigen interaction (data not shown).

In the HA306-318 system, it has been shown that both the spacer length and the length of the oligomer (i.e., number of repetitive epitope units) have a profound effect on the outcome of the T cell response. Testing the SP/2 line with a set of PLP oligomers revealed that also in the PLP system the oligomer length had a similar effect (Fig. 1 B, left). The strongest response was triggered with a 16-mer, whereas the 4-mer, the shortest oligomer tested in this experiment, required 5–10 times higher concentrations. Similar results were also obtained with the T cell clone 8A1 (Fig. 1 B, right). To determine the influence of the spacer on the T cell recognition, this clone was also tested with a synthetic peptide, in which the actual core epitope was extended by parts of the spacer (sp-peptide-sp, see Materials and Methods; Fig. 1 B, right). Although the multimerization of the epitope resulted in a significant increase in antigenicity (>1 log for the 4-mer and >2 logs for the 16-mer), the extension of the epitope by the spacer sequence caused only a slight improvement in the proliferative response. The influence of oligomer length was not evident in lines that did not show an improved response to the oligomers, and the trend was even reversed in clones that recognized oligomers only weakly (e.g., hPLP/c4, data not shown).

T cells that responded most effectively to the stimulation with the 16-mer often showed a reduced proliferation after exposure to the highest 16-mer concentrations (10 or 50 µg/ml). For instance, a maximal proliferative response for the SP/2 (Fig. 1 B, left) and SP/3 lines (Fig. 1 A, top left) or the clone 8A1 (Fig. 1 B, right) or SP/2.2A8 (Fig. 1 A, middle) was triggered at a concentration of ~0.5–1.0 µg/ml 16-mer. The effect resembled high zone suppression and was not seen after incubation with the peptide.

Ex Vivo Response of Primary T Cell Cultures. To determine whether the improved antigenicity, observed for some of the T cells in vitro, would translate into an increased immunogenicity, mice were immunized with the PLP139–151(C140S) peptide, with the 16-mer or, as a control, with adjuvant only (Fig. 2). Primary cell cultures, established from the draining LNs of the primed mice, were then challenged in vitro with titrated amounts of the PLP139–151(C140S) peptide or the 16-mer. PLP139–151 is resticed by I-A^s, and mice from three different strains were used: SJL/J, which are permissive (I-A^s) and EAE susceptible; B10.S, which are permissive (I-A^s) but EAE resistant (30), and BALB/c, which, in principle, are EAE susceptible but are not permissive for this particular epitope (I-A^d).

A specific proliferative response was only observed in the primary cultures derived from SJL/J and B10.S mice treated with antigens (Fig. 2 A, panels 2, 3, 5, and 6). No proliferation was detected in cultures established from BALB/c mice (panels 7–9) and in the control cultures derived from mice primed with adjuvant only (panels 1, 4, and 7). The strength of the T cell response was more vigorous in most cases if the primary culture was stimulated with the 16-mer. This was particularly evident in cultures generated from oligomer-primed mice. Here, often <100-fold lower concentrations of 16-mer than of the peptide were effective (panels 3 and 6). The relative enhancement was more variable in the cultures derived from peptide-primed mice, and frequently these cultures responded equally well to the stimulation by peptide or 16-mer (e.g., Fig. 2 A, panel 2). Cultures derived from mice primed with the 16-mer usually responded strongly to the 16-mer, but in most cases only relatively weakly to the stimulation with the monomeric peptide. The weak response against the peptide might be explained by the predominant stimulation by the 16-mer of low-affinity clones (as suggested by the previous in vitro experiments), whereas the monomer is recognized only by high-affinity clones. In any case, in susceptible SJL mice as well as in resistant B10.S mice, a strong and specific T cell response could be generated by the immunization with the oligomer (panels 3 and 6). The priming with peptide, in particular in B10.S mice (panel 5), usually resulted in weakly responding primary cultures.

No IL-4 was detectable in any of these cultures (not shown). On the other hand, IFN-γ was found in the supernatants of all the primary cell cultures derived from antigen-primed mice, in particular after the challenge with the 16-mer. As an example, the IFN-γ release of the cultures derived from B10.S mice is shown in Fig. 2 B. Although only relatively small amounts (~1 ng/ml) were detected in cultures generated from peptide-primed mice, >6 ng/ml of IFN-γ was measured in the supernatants derived from cultures of 16-mer-primed mice. The relatively high levels of IFN-γ might be indicative of a preferred expansion of Th1 T cells after the immunization with the PLP 16-mer.

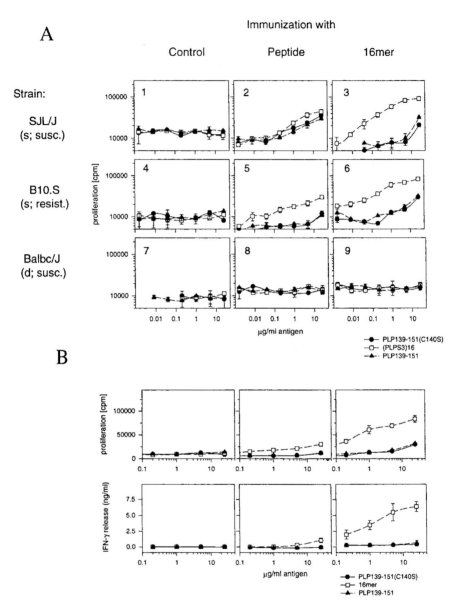

Fig. 2. Ex vivo response of primary LN cultures. (A) Proliferative response of primary LN cultures of mice previously immunized with 50 μg of either the PLP139–151(C140S) peptide (panels 2, 5, and 8) or the 16-mer (panels 3, 6, and 9). Primary LN cultures were prepared from SJL/J mice (panels 1–3), B10.S mice (panels 4–6), and BALB/c mice (panels 7-9). The H2 haplotype and the EAE susceptibility (susc.)/resistance (resist.) of the strains are indicated. The LNCs were isolated 7–12 d after the immunization and challenged in vitro by adding titrated amounts of the unsubstituted PLP139–151 peptide, the PLP139–151(C140S)

In Vivo Effect of PLP139–151(C140S) Oligomers. To determine whether the increased immunogenicity of the oligomer also results in an enhanced encephalitogenicity, a series of in vivo experiments was performed (Fig. 3). After the subcutaneous immunization of SJL/J mice with titrated amounts of either PLP139–151(C140S) peptide or the 16-mer, the mice were observed for the appearance of the typical clinical signs of EAE (fig. 3 A). The score of the clinical symptoms revealed that SJL/J mice were more sensitive to EAE induction with the oligomer than with peptide. Compared with mice immunized with the peptide, they showed an earlier onset and a much more severe progression of the disease. At a dosage of 50 µg, the peptide-primed mice developed EAE on day 13 and had a maximal clinical score of 3.75 (incidence: 3/4, mortality: 75 %). In contrast, the group primed with the 16-mer showed the first signs of the disease almost 4 d earlier (day 9) and reached the maximal clinical score of 5 (i.e., incidence: 4/4; mortality: 100 %). The trend also continued at lower dosages of the antigens. Although at the dosage of 10 µg almost no clinical signs of disease were observed in the group primed with the peptide (incidence: 1/4; mean maximum score: 0.25), 16-mer-primed SJL mice developed a severe disease (incidence: 4/4; onset: day 11.5; mean maximum score: 5; mortality: 100 %). Even at the lowest dosage tested (2 µg), a mild form of EAE was still evident in the group treated with the 16-mer (incidence: 2/4; onset: day 13; mean maximum score: 0,5; mortality: 0 %). At this dosage, no effect was seen in the peptide group.

In the second part of this experiment, we addressed the question as to whether the oligomer could also induce EAE in resistant B10.S mice (Fig. 3 B). In accordance with previous reports (31), no clinical signs of the disease were observed in the B10.S group primed with the peptide. The 16-mer, in contrast, was also encephalitogenic in this strain (no effect with the peptide or the 16-mer was observed in the BALB/c control group). The EAE was only slightly less severe than in SJL/J mice and, at a dosage of 50 µg, induced the disease with an incidence rate of 100 %. Compared with SJL/J mice, in B10.S mice the onset of the disease was delayed by ~3 d and resulted in a mean maximum score of 3.0. CNS immunohistochemistry performed on brain and spinal cord samples of the 16-mer-treated B10.S mice (Fig. 4) revealed an extensive submeningeal,

---

peptide, or the PLP139–151(C140S) 16-mer. As control, the response of cultures derived from mice treated with adjuvant only is shown (panels 1, 4, and 7). (B) Proliferative response (top) and the cytokine release (bottom) of primary LN cultures derived from B10.S mice. The amount of IFN-γ was determined in supernatants taken 96 h after the start of the experiment.

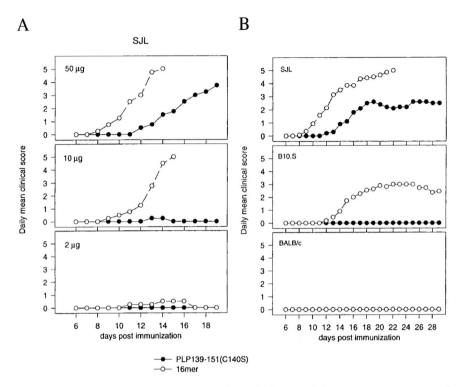

Fig. 3. Induction of EAE with PLP139–151(C140S) oligomer. (A) Dose-response curves of peptide and 16-mer in susceptible SJL/J mice. EAE was induced in groups of four mice by subcutaneous injection of either 50 µg (top), 10 µg (middle), or 2 µg (bottom) of the PLP139-151(C140S) peptide or the 16-mer. The progression of the disease was determined on a daily basis by monitoring the mice for the appearance of clinical symptoms. The severity of the EAE is expressed in the mean score of these symptoms. Four mice per group were used. (B) EAE induction in susceptible and resistant strains. The encephalitogenic effect of 16-mer and peptide was tested with SJL/J mice (permissive/susceptible, top), B10.S mice (permissive/resistant, middle), or BALB/c mice (nonpermissive/susceptible, bottom). The mice were immunized subcutaneously with 50 µg of either the PLP139–151(C140S) peptide or the 16-mer. Filled circles of the peptide-treated BALB/c group are covered by the open symbol of the 16-mer-treated group. The clinical scores respresent a compilation of several experiments using the following numbers of mice: SJL/J, 10 (peptide) and 14 (16-mer); B10.S, 9 (peptide) and 11(16-mer); BALB/c, 6 (peptide) and 8 (16-mer).

perivascular, and parenchymal infiltration (Fig. 4, panel 2), as well as demyelination (panel 4). In contrast, only some minor submeningeal infiltration (panel 1) and no demyelination (panel 3) was detectable in the samples from peptide-primed B10.S mice.

PLP-peptide   PLP-16mer

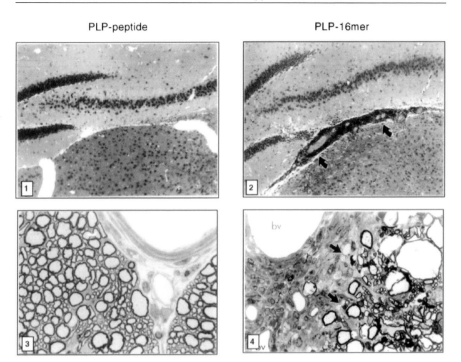

Fig. 4. Pathological analysis of resistent B10.S mice after EAE induction with PLP139–151(C140S) oligomers. B10.S mice were sensitized subcutaneously with 50 µg of either the PLP139–151(C140S) peptide (panels 1 and 3) or the 16-mer (panels 2 and 4). 14 d after disease induction, the animals were perfused with fixative. Paraffin-embedded sections of the brain were stained with hematoxylin and eosin to detect inflammatory infiltrates (panels 1 and 2, original magnifications: ×350), and plastic-embedded sections of the lumbar spinal cord were stained with toluidine blue to detect demyelination (panels 3 and 4, original magnifications: ×750). In animals sensitized with PLP139–151(C140S) peptide, no evidence of inflammation was detected in the brain (panel 1), and no inflammation or demyelination was noted within the spinal cord parenchyma (panel 3). In contrast, in the brains of animals sensitized with the 16-mer, dense accumulations of perivascular cells were observed around vessels overlying the anterior thalamus (arrows, panel 2). In the spinal cord, inflammatory cells were noted around blood vessels (bv), and inflammation, primary demyelination (arrows), and intramyelinic edema were detected within the anterior columns.

To demonstrate that induction of EAE was limited only to permissive strains, mouse strains with various H2 haplotypes were primed with either the peptide or the 16-mer (Table I). In all tested I-A^s-expressing mouse strains, the treatment with the oligomer resulted in the induction of EAE. A.SW, for example, showed symptoms comparable to the ones described for SJL/J. No clinical signs of the disease were observed in mice of the b, d, k, q, and u haplotypes.

Table 1. Clinical EAE in Various Strains of Mice

Mice		Incidence of EAE[1]		Percent disease[2]		Percent mortality[3]		Maximum mean Score[4]		Mean day of onset[4]	
Strain	H2 haplotype	Peptide	16-mer	Peptide	16-mer	Peptide	16-mer	Peptide	16-mer	Peptide	16-mer
SJL/J	s	17/20	14/14	85	100	40	100	3.1±2.0	5.0±0.0	14.0±1.5	10.5±1.2
A.SW	s	5/6	6/6	83	100	66	100	3.5±2.3	5.0±0.0	13.8±2.0	9.8±0.7
B10.S	s	0/9	15/15	0	100	0	33	0	3.1±1.5	–	13.3±3.0
BALB/c	d	0/6	0/8	0	0	0	0	0	0	–	–
B10	b	0/4	0/4	0	0	0	0	0	0	–	–
AKR/J	k	0/4	0/4	0	0	0	0	0	0	–	–
SWR	q	0/4	0/4	0	0	0	0	0	0	–	–
PL/J	u	0/4	0/4	0	0	0	0	0	0	–	–

EAE induction with PLP139–151(C140S) oligomers in different strains of mice. Mice from various strains were immunized with 50 μg of either the PLP139–151(C140S) 16-mer or the peptide as described in Materials and Methods.

[1] Values represent the number of mice with clinical signs of EAE as a fraction of the total number of immunized mice.
[2] Values represent the percentage of immunized mice with clinical signs of disease.
[3] Values representing the percentage of mortality refer to the total number of immunized mice.
[4] Values representing mean day of onset and maximum mean clinical grade were scored as described in reference 28.

In Vivo Effect of MBP86–100 Oligomers. To extend the study to other encephalitogenic T cell epitopes, oligomers were tested in which the PLP139–151(C140S) epitope was replaced by a T cell epitope derived from the MBP protein (MBP86–100). In vitro experiments indicated that, at least in the I-A^s system, MBP86–100 has a significantly lower antigenicity than PLP139–151. T cells, which show an improved response to the oligomer, seem to be less frequent in SJL mice and the ex vivo experiments revealed less impressive results compared with the PLP139–151 system (data not shown). However, to test if MBP86–100 oligomers showed some enhanced encephalitogenicity, the same series of in vivo experiments was performed as described previously for the PLP oligomers (Fig. 5).

The MBP86–100 16-mer was found to be a fairly potent inducer of EAE. Compared with the effect of the peptide, the application of the 16-mer resulted in an earlier onset and more severe progression of the disease. In a dose-response study with SJL/J mice (Fig. 5, left), disease induction with the peptide was only observed after an injection of 100 μg, the highest dosage used in this experiment (incidence: 2/4, onset: 13.5, maximal mean score: 1.7, mortality: 0 %). One third of this amount, 33 μg, was insufficient to trigger EAE. In contrast, the effect of the MBP86–100 16-mer was significantly stronger. At a dosage of 100 μg, all of the SJL mice treated with the 16-mer developed a fatal disease (incidence: 4/4, onset: 10.7, maximal mean score: 5.0, mortality: 100 %). The encephalitogenic effect decreased at 33 μg (incidence: 3/4, onset: 13.6, maximal mean score: 2.75, mortality: 50 %) but was still evident at a dosage of 11 μg where some cases of mild forms of EAE were observed (incidence: 2/4, onset: day 16.5, maximal mean score: 0.75, mortality: 0 %). Importantly, it was also possible to induce EAE in B10.S mice (Fig. 5, right). Compared with the PLP139–151 system, the effect of the MBP86–100 16-mer was weaker but 50 μg of the antigen was stil sufficient to induce the disease in the majority of the tested animals (incidence: 3/5; onset: day 18; maximal mean score: 1.6; mortality: 20 %). The same treatment with the peptide did not cause any effect.

Effect of Intravenous Administration of Oligomers on the Progression of EAE.
To examine whether the oligomers could have a potential therapeutic impact in the suppression of EAE, mice were treated by intravenous injection with PBS solutions of the PLP139–151(C140S) antigens (Fig. 6). The experiment was carried out in SJL/J mice in which the disease was induced by the subcutaneous administration of 50 μg PLP139–151(C140S) peptide in CFA. The mice were treated either before (days –7 and –3; Fig. 6, left) or after the disease induction (days 3 and 7; Fig. 6, right). The animals received the intravenous injections of peptide (top) or 16-mer (bottom) at a dosage of 50 μg, and control groups received a mock treatment with PBS.

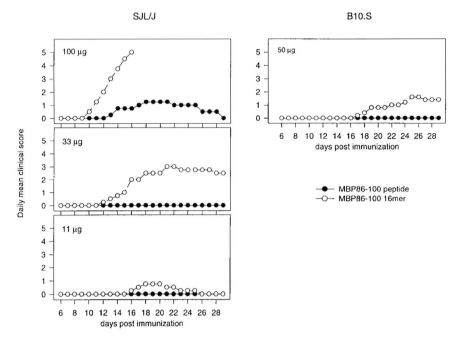

Fig. 5. Induction of EAE with MBP86–100 oligomers. Clinical scores of mice treated subcutaneously with MBP86–100 peptide or MBP86–100 16-mer. The experiment was carried out as described in the legend to Fig. 3. The SJL/J and B10.S mice received the amounts of antigens indicated in the figure. Four mice per group were used in these experiments.

The intravenous treatment with the 16-mer almost completely prevented the development of the disease (Fig. 6, bottom). With the treatment before the disease induction (bottom left), four of the five mice did not show any clinical signs, and only one mouse developed a very mild form of EAE (score of 1, resulting in a mean score of 0.2). Importantly, the effect of the 16-mer was also evident if the treatment was done several days after the induction of the disease (bottom right). Two injections of 50 µg were sufficient to reduce the maximal mean clinical score to a value of 1.3 compared with a score of 4.5 in the control group. After the initial attack, which peaked at day 19, most of the mice returned within 6 d to a condition virtually free of any clinical symptoms. In contrast to the treatment with the 16-mer, the effect of the peptide was far less dramatic. Although peptide treatment before the disease induction (Fig. 6, top left) resulted at least in some reduction of the severity of the EAE progression (maximal mean score of 2.2), the treatment after disease induction (top right) resulted

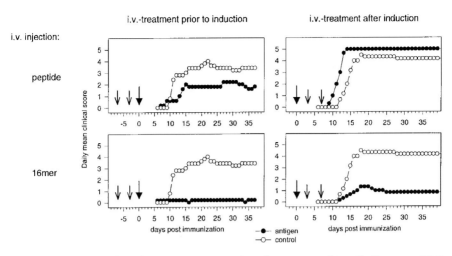

Fig. 6. Suppression of EAE by intravenous injection of PLP139–151(C140S) oligomers. SJL/J mice were treated with intravenous injection of either PLP139–152(C140S) peptide (top) or the 16-mer (bottom) seveal days before (left) or after (right) disease induction. EAE was induced by a subcutaneous injection of 50 μg PLP139–151(C140S) peptide emulsified in CFA (filled arrowhead). The mice received the intravenous injections of peptide or 16-mer on the day indicated by small open arrows. The daily mean clinical scores of the mice treated intravenously with antigens are shown in comparison to the score of control groups, which received mock intravenous injections of PBS instead of antigen. Groups of five or six mice were used for the experiments. The incidence rates were determined as 5/5 (control), 5/5 (peptide), and 2/5 (16-mer) for the groups treated before the disease induction and as 6/6 (control), 6/6 (peptide), and 4/6 (16-mer) for the groups treated after the disease induction.

in acceleration of disease progression. The onset shifted by almost 2 d, and a maximal mean score of 5 (i.e., 100 % mortality) was reached earlier, by day 14.

The effect of peptide treatment on enhancing instead of suppressing the disease progression could not be overcome by an increase in dosage. Even when 250 μg was administered to the animals, no reverse in the trend was apparent (data not shown). On the other hand, with the 16-mer a single injection of 50 μg on day 7 was found to be sufficient to produce a strong suppression (Fig. 7, bottom). At this time point, only very little submeningeal, perivascular infiltration was evident in brain sections taken from SJL/J mice immunized with the peptide (data not shown). However, the effect of the 16-mer was found to be highly specific, and no suppression was evident if the disease was induced with the PLP178–191 peptide (Fig. 7, top) instead of the PLP139–151 peptide (Fig. 7, bottom). Similar results were also obtained with MBP antigens containing the epitopes MBP86–100 and MBP86–101 (Fig. 8). Only a relatively modest sup-

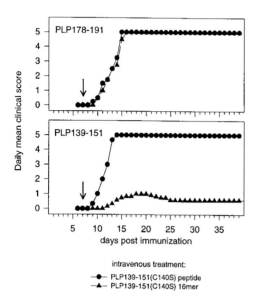

Fig. 7. Specificity of EAE suppression by intravenous injections of PLP139–151(C140S) 16-mers. SJL/L mice received intravenous injections of 50 µg PLP139–151(C140S) peptide or PLP 139–151(C140S) 16-mer 7 d after the induction of the disease by the subcutaneous injection of 50 µg PLP178–191(C183S) (top) or PLP139–151(C140S) peptide (bottom). Groups of six mice were used for the experiment. The incidence rates were determined as 6/6 (peptide) and as 6/6 (16-mer) for the groups immunized with the PLP178–191(C183S) peptide and as 6/6 (peptide) and 4/6 (16-mer) for the groups immunized with the PLP139–151(C140S) peptide.

pression was observed after an injection of 100 µg of MBP86–100 16-mer on days 3 and 7 (triangles, top). The effect was greatly enhanced after using a 16-mer containing the more antigenic epitope MBP86–101 at an increased dosage (200 µg) on days 8 and 12. Also in the MBP system, the intravenous treatment with peptides had little or no effect (Filled circles).

Ex vivo experiments with primary LN cultures (LNCs) further indicated that in mice treated with the PLP139–151(C140S) 16-mer, the specific response against this antigen was either reduced, or, as shown in the top left panel of Fig. 9 (triangles), completely absent. In contrast, the antigen-specific response of LNCs from peptide-treated mice (filled circles) was similar to that of the control group (open circles). This silencing of the T cell response, presumably due to apoptosis or anergy induction, was found to be antigen specific, since the T cell proliferation triggered by staphylococcal enterotoxin A or B was

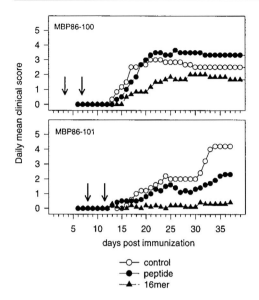

Fig. 8. Suppression of EAE by intravenous injections of oligomers containing the MBP86–100 epitope. SJL/J mice were treated with intravenous injections if MBP86–100 (top) or MBP86–101 (bottom). EAE was induced on day 0 by the subcutaneous injection of 100 µg MBP86–100 or 200 µg MBP86–101 peptide, respectively. The mice were treated intravenously with peptide, 16-mer, or PBS at the indicated time points (arrows) and received dosages of 100 µg of the MBP86–100 or 200 µg of the MBP86–101 antigens. Groups of 5–10 mice were used for the experiment. The incidence rates were determined as 5/6 (control), 6/6 (peptide), and 4/6 (16-mer) for the groups primed and treated with the MBP86–100 epitope and as 5/5 (control), 9/10 (peptide), and 4/10 (16-mer) for the groups primed and treated with the MBP86–101 epitope.

unaffected (not shown). The histological analysis of the tissues taken from the mice revealed interesting differences in the pathology between the three groups. In the mock-treated animals (Fig. 9, top right), the lesions showed prominent demyelination (arrowheads) in the presence of an inflammatory infiltrate that contained numerous polymorphonuclear cells (small arrows). In the peptide-treated animals (bottom left), inflammation and demyelination were also evident and the lesions contained mostly mononuclear cells. Importantly, however, in cord tissue from animals tolerized with the 16-mer no inflammation or demyelination was noted (bottom right), although a low level of inflammation was still present in the brains of these animals (data not shown).

Long-Term Effects, Control of Relapse, and Induction with Spinal Cord. Without the 16-mer treatment, in most cases the mice did not recover from the initial

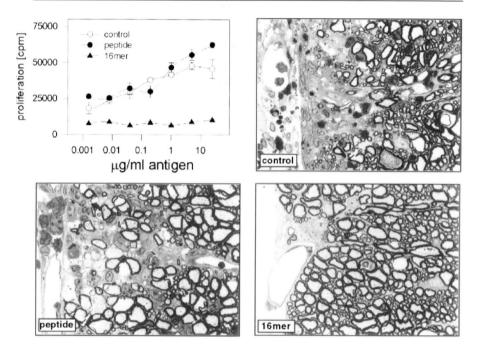

Fig. 9. Pathological analysis and lymphocyte proliferative response after intravenous treatment with PLP139-151(C140S) 16-mer. EAE was induced in SJL/J mice with PLP139-151(C140S) peptide. 7 d later, the mice received intravenous injections of either 50 μg PLP139-151(C140S) peptide, PLP139-151(C140S) 16-mer, or mock injections of PBS. 7 d later (day 14), LNs were removed to test the ex vivo response, and the mice were perfused with Trump's fixative before the removal of the spinal cord for the histological analysis of disease. The ex vivo response of primary LNCs of peptide-, 16-mer-, and mock-treated mice is shown in the top left panel. LNCs were challenged in a proliferation assay with titrated amounts of PLP139-151(C140S) 16-mer (top left). The proliferation assay was performed essentially as described in the legend to Fig. 2. The other panels show the histochemical image of 1-μm-thick plastic-embedded tissue stained with toluidine blue. The samples derived from the mock-treated control animal (top right) and from the peptide-treated ouse (bottom left) show submeningeal lesions typical of EAE (meninges located on the left of the panels). The meningeal vessels were inflamed, and numerous inflammatory cells were detected within the cord parenchyma (arrows). In tissues from control animals, large numbers of polymorphonuclear cells were evident (small arrows). Demyelinated axons (arrowheads) were present within the inflamed area of the cord. In contrast, in the sample derived from the 16-mer-treated mouse (bottom right), the meningeal vessels were not inflamed and the cord parenchyma showed no evidence of inflammation or demyelination. Original magnifications: ×500.

attack, whereas with the 16-mer treatment the disease was suppressed for at least 40 d. Long-terms studies revealed that after that period the mice started to relapse (Fig. 10 A, top). The time frame between the acute episode and the relapse is consistent with the appearance of a new wave of autoreactive PLP139–151-specific T cells from the thymus. Although during the relapsing phase the T cell response reportedly becomes more heterogeneous due to epitope spreading (32–34), an additional intravenous injection with the PLP139–151(C140S) 16-mer on day 40 was still effective in further preventing the appearance of clinical symptoms (Fig. 10 A, bottom). A similar suppression was also achieved when the disease was triggered by broadly stimulating spinal cord homogenate instead of a single epitope (Fig. 10 B). Compared with mice induced with the PLP139–151 peptide, the treatment was slightly less effective, but a strong suppression was also evident after induction with spinal cord (Fig. 10 B, top). Previous reports indicated that PLP139–151 is the dominant epitope in SJL/J mice after immunization with spinal cord homogenate (35). By using a 16-mer with this immunodominant epitope the maximal daily mean score of the initial attack was reduced to only 1.7 compared with 4.5 for the control group, and a complete recovery of the 16-mer-treated mice was observed by day 34 before the mice started to relapse. A second dose, administered on day 12, greatly enhanced the suppressive effect (Fig. 10 B, bottom). In this experiment, the mice treated twice with the 16-mer remained free of clinical symptoms for >60 d.

Discussion

The trimolecular interaction of TCR–peptide–MHC represents the structural basis of the immune response. Several attempts have already been made to modulate this interaction with the intent to enhance the response to a vaccine (36–38), and multimerization or oligomerization is another approach in this direction. Soluble multivalent peptide–MHC complexes were previously shown to simultaneously engage multiple TCRs resulting in complexes, which are significantly more stable than the respective monomeric complex (39, 40). Furthermore, the TCR cross-linking promoted by this interaction initiates signal transduction and triggers the activation cascade of the T cell, which significantly lowers the threshold for the activation (41). In addition, the use of multimerized T cell epitopes can produce similar effects. The multimerized antigens, which were designed to form multivalent arrays of peptide–MHC complexes on the surface of the APCs, can show, in some cases, great enhancement in the antigenicity of the epitope.

A

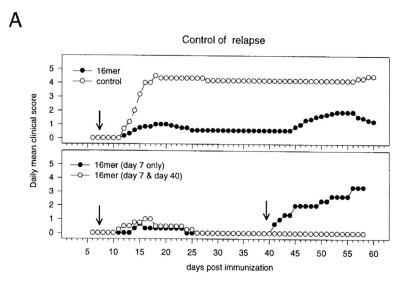

B

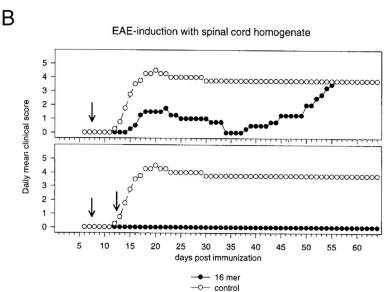

Fig. 10. Control of relapse and effect of intravenous treatment with PLP139-151(C140S) 16-mer after EAE induction with spinal cord homogenate. (A) Long-term effect of the treatment with PLP 16-mer and prevention of relapse. The top panel shows an experiment in which SJL/J mice received only a single intravenous dosage of 50 μg PLP139-151(C140S) 16-mer on day 7. The clinical score is plotted in comparison to the score of a control group treated with PBS only. In the experiment shown in the bottom panel, mice either received only the single dosage of 50 μg 16-mer on day 7 or were treated again the same way on day 40. Groups of four mice were used for the experiments, and the disease was induced by

The oligomerized encephalitogenic antigens presented in this study were not only more effective in the stimulation of antigen-specific T cells in vitro, but also induced stronger primary T cell responses in vivo. The priming of mice with these antigens resulted in the manifestation of very severe forms of EAE, evident even in resistant strains. Earlier studies suggested that the failure of resistant B10.S mice to develop EAE is caused by a paucity of high-affinity autoreactive T cells (42, 43). Since the oligomerized antigens were particularly effective in the stimulation of low-avidity T cells, the increased encephalitogenicity might be attributable to the induction of a broader T cell response by the recruitment of a larger number of T cell clones. Part of this might be due to a potentially reduced need for costimulatory signals. Studies with tetrameric peptide–MHC complexes indicated that at least for these tetramers the influence of CD4 on the binding is diminished (40). In addition, the activation of the APCs by MHC cross-linking (1, 44) and the "proteinization" of the epitope could contribute to the effect. An increased stability of the epitope, altered routes of antigen presentation, and a more effective T cell stimulation by an activated APC might be relevant particularly for the increase in antigenicity in vivo. Another factor might be the strong enhancement of a Th1-type T cell response. Autoreactive $CD4^+$ T cells of the Th1 type are the driving force in T cell-mediated autoimmune diseases, and a preferred activation of this T cell subset would certainly promote the progression of EAE. In fact, a recent study (45) indicated that the resistance of B10.S mice might be due to a failure of antigen-specific $CD4^+$ T cells to upregulate CD40 ligand. This failure abrogates the release of IL-12 and subsequently affects the expression level of the $\beta2$ subunit of IL-12R, a receptor crucial in controlling Th1 lineage commitment. At this point, however, it is not clear whether the enhancement of encephalitogenicity is actually caused by a selective activation of Th1 T cells.

Maybe even more important than the improved stimulation is the effect of oligomerized antigens if administered intravenously on the suppression of the autoimmune disease. High zone tolerance as a mechanism of T cell tolerization has been known for some time (13), but its practicality has been limited by the requirement of extremely high antigen (peptide, protein) levels. The enhanced antigenicity of multimerized antigens might make this approach more feasible.

◀———————————————————————————————

subcutaneous administration of PLP139-151(C140S) peptide. (B) Treatment of EAE with PLP139-151(C140S) 16-mer after induction with spinal cord homogenate. The experiment was carried out as described above except that 4 mg of spinal cord homogenate instead of the PLP peptide was used for the disease induction. The SJL/J mice received intravenous injections of 50 µg 16-mer either on day 8 (top) or on days 8 and 12 (bottom). The control group was treated with mock injections of PBS. Groups of five mice were used for this experiment.

A drastic decrease in incidence and severity of EAE was achieved after a single intravenous treatment with a relatively low dosage of 50 µg per mouse. In vitro experiments with HA306–318 oligomers and human influenza virus–specific T cells indicated that the underlying mechanism is most likely the apoptotic elimination of the "overstimulated" autoreactive T cell (data not shown). The reduction in the antigen-specific ex vivo response of mice treated with encephalitogenic oligomers and the long period of protection after treatment are consistent and suggest that this mechanism is also responsible for the specific suppression in the EAE system. Importantly, the suppression was also observed at the onset of the relapsing phase and after disease induction with spinal cord homogenate. The effectiveness of the oligomers in these situations together with the observation that a fraction of the autoreactive T cell population actually fails to respond to the multimerized antigen suggests that, in addition to the antigen-specific suicidal T cell elimination, "bystander" effects contribute to the high zone suppression.

Thus, oligomerized antigens can be effective in the induction and suppression of the immune response. In addition to their use as vaccines for the stimulation of preventive pathogen-specific T cell responses, they might be particularly valuable for the immunotherapy of tumors. Most chronic autoimmune diseases are mediated by $CD4^+$ T cells, and the recruitment of autoreactive $CD4^+$ T cells specific for tumor antigens (46) might permit the developemt of a similar situation, with the immune response directed towards the specific destruction of the transformed tissue. Furthermore, the striking effects of multimeric T cell epitopes in high zone applications might provide a new stimulus for the use of autoantigens in therapies aimed at the specific suppression of acute or chronic autoimmune states.

We are very grateful to S. Jah and M.L. Wong for excellent technical assistance, and to K. Wormstadt for animal maintenance. In particular, we thank M. Lenardo for thoroughly reviewing the manuscript and for his helpful comments.

This research was supported by National Institute of Health grants 5R35-CA47554 and N01-AI45198.

Acknowledgement

The permission for the reproduction of the Journal of Experimental Medicine (The Rockefeller University Press) 2000, Vol. 191, 717–730, is gratefully acknowledged.

References

1. Rötzschke O, Falk K, Strominger JL (1997) Superactivation of an immune response triggered by oligomerized T cell epitopes. Proc Natl Acad Sci USA 94:14642–14647
2. Martin R and McFarland H (1996) Experimental immunotherapies for multiple sclerosis. Springer Semin Immunopathol 18:1–24
3. McFarlin DE, Blank SE, Kibler RF, McKneally S, Shapira R (1973) Experimental allergic encephalomyelitis in the rat: response to encephalitogenic proteins and peptides. Science 179:478–480
4. Tuohy VK, Lu Z, Sobel RA, Laursen RA, Lees MB (1989) Identification of an encephalitogenic determinant of myelin proteolipid protein for SJL mice. J Immunol 142:1523–1527
5. Greer JM, Kuchroo VK, Sobel RA, Lees MB (1992) Identification and characterization of a second encephalitogenic determinant of myelin proteolipid protein (residues 178–191) for SJL mice. J Immunol 149:783–788
6. Zamvil SS, Mitchell DJ, Moore AC, Kitamura K, Steinmann L, Rothbard JB (1986) T-cell epitope of the autoantigen myelin basic protein that induces encephalomyelitis. Nature 324:258–260
7. Kono DH, Urban JL, Horvath SJ, Ando DG, Saavedra RA, Hood L (1988) Two minor determinants of myelin basic protein induce experimental allergic encephalomyelitis in SJL/J mice. J Exp Med 168:213–227
8. Mendel I, Kerlero de Rosbo N, Ben-Nun A (1995) A myelin oligodendrocyte glycoprotein peptide induces typical chronic experimental autoimmune encephalomyelitis in H-2b mice: fine specificity and T cell receptor V beta expression of encephalitogenic T cells. Eur J Immunol 25:1951–1959
9. Butterfield RJ, Blankenhorn EP, Roper RJ, Zachary JF, Doerge RW, Sudweeks J, Rose J, Teuscher C (1999) Genetic analysis of disease subtypes and sexual dimorphisms in mouse experimental allergic encephalomyelitis (EAE): relapsing/remitting and monophasic remitting/nonrelapsing EAE are immunogenetically distinct. J Immunol 162:3096–3102
10. Segal BM, Shevach EM (1996) IL-12 unmasks latent autoimmune disease in resistant mice. J Exp Med 184:771–775
11. Santambrogio L, Crisi GM, Leu J, Hochwald GM, Ryan T, Thorbecke GJ (1995) Tolerogenic forms of autoantigens and cytokines in the induction of resistance to experimental allergic encephalomyelitis. J Neuroimmunol 58: 211–222
12. Leonard JP, Waldburger KE, Goldman SJ (1995) Prevention of experimental autoimmune encephalomyelitis by antibodies against interleukin 12. J Exp Med 181:381–386
13. Diener E, Feldmann M (1972) Mechanisms at the cellular level during induction of high zone tolerance in vitro. Cell Immunol 5:130–136
14. Gaur A, Wiers B, Liu A, Rothbard J, Fathman CG (1992) Amelioration of autoimmune encephalomyelitis by myelin basic protein synthetic peptide-induced anergy. Science 258:1491–1494

15. Critchfield JM, Racke MK, Zuniga-Pflucker JC, Cannella B, Raine CS, Goverman J, Lenardo MJ (1994) T cell deletion in high antigen dose therapy of autoimmune encephalomyelitis. Science 263:1139–1143

16. Whitacre CC, Gienapp IE, Meyer A, Cox KL, Javed N (1996) Treatment of autoimmune disease by oral tolerance to autoantigens. Clin Immunol Immunopathol 80:S31–S39

17. Kennedy KJ, Smith WS, Miller SD, Karpus WJ (1997) Induction of antigen-specific tolerance for the treatment of ongoing, relapsing autoimmune encephalomyelitis: a comparison between oral and peripheral tolerance. J Immunol 159:1036–1044

18. Weiner HL (1997) Oral tolerance: immune mechanisms and treatment of autoimmune diseases. Immunol Today 18:335–343

19. Liu JQ, Bai XF, Shi FD, Xiao BG, Li HL, Levi M, Mustafa M, Wahren B, Link H (1998) Inhibition of experimental autoimmune encephalomyelitis in Lewis rats by nasal administration of encephalitogenic MBP peptides: synergistic effects of MBP 68–86 and 87–99. Int Immunol 10:1139–1148

20. Tonegawa SMS (1997) Tolerance induction and autoimmune encephalomyelitis amelioration after administration of myelin basic protein–derived peptide. J Exp Med 186:507–515

21. Staykova MA, Simmons RD, Willenborg DO (1997) Infusion of soluble myelin basic protein protects longterm against induction of experimental autoimmune encephalomyelitis. Immunol Cell Biol 75:54–64

22. St Louis J, Zhang XM, Heber-Katz E, Uniyal S, Robbinson D, Singh B, Strejan GH (1999) Tolerance induction by acylated peptides: effect on encephalitogenic T cell lines. J Autoimmun 12:177–189

23. Brocke S, Gijbels K, Allegretta M, Ferber I, Piercy C, Blankenstein T, Martin R, Utz U, Karin N, Mitchell D (1996) Treatment of experimental encephalomyelitis with a peptide analogue of myelin basic protein [published erratum at 392:630) Nature 379:343–346

24. Elliott EA, Cofiell R, Wilkins JA, Raine CS, Matis LA, Mueller JP (1997) Immune tolerance mediated by recombinant proteolipid protein prevents experimental autoimmune encephalomyelitis. J Neuroimmunol 79:1–11

25. Elliott EA, McFarland HI, Nye SH, Cofiell R, Wilson TM, Wilkins JA, Squinto SP, Matis LA, Mueller JP (1996) Treatment of experimental encephalomyelitis with a novel chimeric fusion protein of myelin basic protein and proteolipid protein. J Clin Invest 98:1602–1612

26. Min B, Legge KL, Pack C, Zaghouani H (1998) Neonatal exposure to a self-peptide-immunoglobulin chimera circumvents the use of adjuvant and confers resistance to autoimmune disease by a novel mechanism involving interleukin 4 lymph node derivation and interferon γ-mediated splenic anergy. J Exp Med 188:2007–2017

27. Leadbetter EA, Bourque CR, Devaux B, Olson CD, Sunshine GH, Hirani S, Wallner BP, Smilek DE, Happ MP (1998) Experimental autoimmune encephalomyelitis induced with a combination of myelin basic protein and myelin oligodendrocyte glycoprotein is ameliorated by administration of a single myelin basic protein peptide. J Immunol 161:504–512

28. Santambrogio L, Hochwald GM, Saxena B, Leu CH, Martz JE, Carlino JA, Ruddle NH, Palladino MA, Gold LI, Thorbecke GJ (1993) Studies in the mechanisms by which transforming growth factor-beta (TGF-beta) protects against allergic ence-

phalomyelitis. Antagonism between TGF-beta and tumor necrosis factor. J Immunol 151:1116–1127

29. Santambrogio L, Lee MB, Sobel RA (1998) Altered peptide ligand modulation of experimental allergic encephalomyelitis: immune responses within the CNS. J Neuroimmunol 81:1–13

30. Lublin FD, Knobler RL, Doherty PC, Korngold R (1986) Relapsing experimental allergic encephalomyelitis in radiation bone marrow chimeras between high and low susceptible strains of mice. Clin Exp Immunol 66:491–496

31. Encinas JA, Lees MB, Sobel RA, Symonowicz C, Greer JM, Shovlin CL, Weiner HL, Seidmann CE, Seidmann JG, Kuchroo VK (1996) Genetic analysis of susceptibility to experimental autoimmune encephalomyelitis in a cross between SJL/J and B10.S mice. J Immunol 157:2186–2192

32. Lehmann PV, Forsthuber T, Miller A, Sercarz EE (1992) Spreading of T-cell autoimmunity to cryptic determinants of an autoantigen. Nature 358:155–157

33. McRae BL, Vanderlugt CL, Dal Canto MC, Miller SD (1995) Functional evidence for epitope spreading in the relapsing pathology of experimental autoimmune encephalomyelitis. J Exp Med 182:75–85

34. Tuohy VK, Yu M, Yin L, Kawczak JA, Johnson JM, Mathisen PM, Weinstock-Guttman B, Kinkel RP (1998) The epitope spreading cascade during progression of experimental autoimmune encephalomyelitis and multiple sclerosis. Immunol Rev 164:93–100

35. Whitham RH, Bourdette DN, Hashim GA, Herndon RM, Ilg RC, Vandenbark AA, Offner H (1991) Lymphocytes from SJL/J mice immunized with spinal cord respond selectively to a peptide of proteolipid protein and transfer relapsing demyelinating experimental autoimmune encephalomyelitis. J Immunol 146:101–107

36. Corradin G, Demitz S (1997) Peptide-MHC complexes assembled following multiple pathways: an opportunity for the design of vaccines and therapeutic molecules. Hum Immunol 54:137–147

37. Barber BH (1997) The immunotargeting approach to adjuvant-independent subunit vaccine design. Semin Immunol 9:293–301

38. Urban RG, Chicz RM, Hedley ML (1997) The discovery and use of HLA-associated epitopes as drugs. Crit Rev Immunol 17:387–397

39. Altman JD, Moss PAH, Goulder PJR, Barouch DH, McHeyzer-Williams MG, Bell JI, McMichael AJ, Davis MM (1996) Phenotypic analysis of antigen-specific T lymphocytes [published erratum at 280:1821] Science 274:94–96

40. Crawford F, Kozono H, White J, Marrack P, Kappler J (1998) Detection of antigen-specific T cells with multivalent soluble class II MHC covalent peptide complexes. Immunity 8:675–682

41. Boniface JJ, Rabinowitz JD, Wulfing C, Hampl J, Reich Z, Altmann JD, Kantor, Beeson C, Mc Connell HM, Davis MM (1998) Initiation of signal transduction through the T cell receptor requires the multivalent engagement of peptide/MHC ligands [published erratum at 9:891]. Immunity 9:459–466

42. Binder TA, Greiner DL, Grunnet M, Goldschneider I (1993) Relative susceptibility of SJL/J and B10.S mice to experimental allergic encephalomyelitis (EAE) is determined by the ability of prethymic cells in bone marrow to develop into EAE effector T cells. J Neuroimmunol 42:23–32

43. Binder TA, Clark RB, Goldschneider I (1991) Relative susceptibility of SJL/J and B10.S mice to experimental allergic encephalomyelitis is correlated with high and low responsiveness to myelin basic protein. J Neuroimmunol 35:31–43
44. Mehindate K, Thibodeau J, Dohlsten M, Kalland T, Sekaly RP, Mourad W (1995) Cross-linking of major histocompatibility complex class II molecules by staphylococcal enterotoxin A superantigen is a requirement for inflammatory cytokine gene expression. J Exp Med 182:1573–1577
45. Chang JT, Shevach EM, Segal BJ (1999) Regulation of interleukin(IL)-1212 receptor β2 subunit expression by endogenous IL-12: a critical step in the differentiation of pathogenic autoreactive T cells. J Exp Med 189:969–978
46. Topalian SL, Gonazles MI, Parkhurst M, Li YF, Southwood S, Sette A, Rosenberg SA, Robbins PF (1996) Melanoma-specific CD4+ T cells recognize nonmutated HLA-DR-restricted tyrosinase epitopes. J Exp Med 183:1965–1971

Determination of the Expressed T cell Repertoire: The Outcome of Competition at the Levels of Antigen Presentation and T cell Receptor Recognition

E. Maverakis[1], J. Beech, H. Deng, C. Schneider, P. van den Elzen, T. Madakamutil, F. Ria, K. Moudgil, V. Kumar, A. Campagnoni, and E.E. Sercarz

The first half of the 20th century saw a revelation in our understanding of the exquisite specificity of antibodies, best exemplified in the work by Karl Landsteiner. A single substituent on a hapten could be readily distinguished from a closely related one by an animal's antiserum. The various antibodies in that antiserum, with their unique perspectives of these cross-reactive haptens/determinants, combined to provide an unmistakable portrait of each region of the antigen. Of course, some antibodies overlapped with others so that, in a sense, a continuum of antibody footprints could be drawn covering the structure.

The nature of T cell specificity was first evident in descriptions of cross-reactivity in delayed hypersensitivity (1). Denatured proteins and native forms cross-reacted, whereas at the B cell level, linear determinants failed to cross-react with assembled determinants, found to be dependent on the tertiary structure of the antigen. This was understood when it became clear that tightly-folded proteins had to become unfolded and then bound to MHC molecules for presentation to T cells (2). Furthermore, for class I binding, it proved necessary for short peptides (8–10-mers) to be processed from the native molecule. Eventually, X-ray crystallography revealed that each MHC molecule had a unique peptide binding groove (3–6), allowing binding of peptides complementary to its pockets and folds. The T cell receptor's footprint on this MHC-peptide ligand complex included antigenic residues protruding from the MHC groove as well as from the helices of the MHC molecule itself (7–10).

[1] La Jolla Institute for Allergy and Immunology, 10355 Science Center Drive, San Diego, California 92121

Competition at the Level of Binding to MHC Class II Molecules

While the short class I-binding peptides are firmly attached at each end to charged residues of the MHC, the class II-binding peptides can be of variable size (11) since the ends of the MHC class II groove are open (6), permitting the peptide to bind while still part of the native or partially fragmented antigen (12, 13). Initially, it was thought that the most probable fate of a protein antigen during its processing involved a proteolytic reduction to the peptide level, followed by binding within the vesicular compartment to a class II molecule. However, increasing evidence has pointed to a more probable mechanism in which a large fragment of the antigen (13), or the partially unfolded whole molecule itself (12, 14), binds to the class II molecule, protecting the groove-bound peptide from proteolytic cleavage (15, 16), while the flanking long overhangs outside the MHC groove are subjected to both endopeptidic and exopeptidic enyzme attack. The possibility thus arises that as the antigen becomes unfolded, different MHC molecules will compete for binding to the first available stretch of the antigen displaying a determinant (17). The winning MHC will bind to the most available affine determinant protecting it from enzymatic degradation. This competition for "determinant capture" dictates that only a small number of determinants will be competitively favored for presentation to T cells.

The Initial Processing of a Tightly Folded Antigen

A tightly-folded molecule such as hen egg lysozyme (HEL) cannot be cleaved readily until it is partially denatured, which enables an endopeptidase to make the first nick in its structure. The identity of such endopeptidases that make the first cleavage has been a mystery until recently when two different approaches yielded two possible candidates. Manoury, Watts and their colleagues isolated an asparagine-specific cysteine endopeptidase (18). In studying the antigen processing of a domain of the microbial tetanus toxin antigen (TTCF), it was discovered that the cleavage by the asparagine-specific cysteine endopeptidase was required for the successful presentation of TTCF to a panel of TTCF-specific T cell clones (18). Using another approach, Schneider et al., found that by mutating HEL to introduce a dibasic processing site adjacent to a subdominant determinant, the determinant's ability to be presented was enhanced 10–40 fold (19). This suggests that transformations of processing sites on immunologically relevant molecules (self molecules with the ability of inducing autoimmunity or tumor immunity) could have crucial consequences.

We imagine that Karl Landsteiner might have been excited by the idea of changing a single residue on a protein to achieve a profound result.

Readily Processed and Poorly Processed Antigenic Determinants

Originally the concept of crypticity was established with the use of T cell proliferation assays. As the first studies of T cell responses to intact antigens revealed very focused responses (20–24), limited to a few or to a single region, the belief arose that holes in the T cell repertoire were prevalent. While examples of holes in the repertoire exist (25, 26), we favored the idea that a primary consideration for immunodominance was the competitive nature of the processing and presentational events. Dominant determinants were defined as the regions of the molecule readily processed by the APC (27). In contrast, cryptic determinants were defined as those poorly displayed after processing. Although cryptic determinants are not readily processed from within the context of the native protein, when provided in the form of a peptide, they can induce a response. To date several additional criteria and reasons for crypticity have been proposed (26, 28, 29).

Determinant display hierarchies have now been confirmed by direct elution experiments. Unanue and colleagues endogenously expressed HEL and then eluted the processed peptides from the surface of APCs (30), showing that relatively few regions of the intact molecule are presented by the APC. Moreover, each determinant consists of a family of overlapping peptides with the same core determinant but with flanking regions of differing lengths (31). In our laboratory, we have obtained similar results by using T cell hybridomas as detectors of determinant display. Although this system does not provide information on the identity of naturally processed peptides, it can sensitively portray differences in responsiveness to all the members within a determinant envelope and in this way provide estimates of determinant display (32, 33).

Determinant Capture:
The Establishment of Determinant Display Hierarchies

The first direct demonstration of determinant capture occurred in comparing the HEL-specific T cell determinant structure in NOD and (NOD × BALB/c) F1 animals (Figure 1). It was known that BALB/c animals when primed with whole HEL respond to a single dominant determinant, p106–116 (34). When HEL was used to prime NOD animals, two non-overlapping determinants induced responses, included within peptides 13–25 and 91–105. However

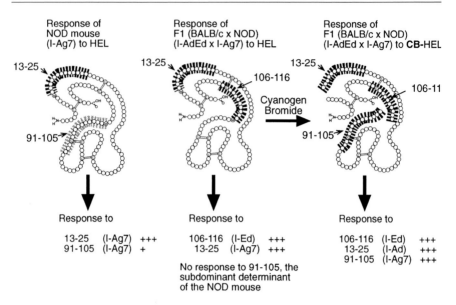

Fig. 1. In the response to HEL by the NOD mouse with its I-Ag7 molecule, peptide 13–25 is dominant, whereas peptide 91–105 gives a subdominant response. In order to study possible determinant capture by the very dominant 106–116/Ed determinant, the F1 between BALB/c and NOD was produced and the response to HEL was again studied. As predicted, there remained no response whatever to 91–105 in the F1, presumably owing to the existence of the neighboring 106–116 and its capture by I-Ed. In order to test this notion, cyanogen bromide treatment of HEL was employed, since it cleaves HEL at the C-terminal side of methionine residues at aa 12 and 105. The latter cleavage separates 106–116 from 91–105 so that they can be independently bound to their corresponding MHC molecules. Indeed, when this molecule (CB-HEL) was used as the immunogen, not only was the response to 91–105 revealed but because of its enhanced access, this response became a dominant one. Accordingly, the lack of response to 91–105 after HEL immunization of the F1 was not due to a regulatory effect or the lack of T cells or of APC function, but rather to the determinant capture effect by I-Ed.

(NOD × BALB/c) F1 animals responded only to 106–116 and to 11–25 (17). Presumably, determinant capture of the 106–116 region by I-E^d prevented the display of the contiguous 91–105 determinant by I-A^{g7} in the F1 animals. Since competition amongst MHC class II molecules requires determinants to reside on the adjacent stretch of protein, cleaving of the antigen to divide one determinant from its competitor should allow for the presentation of both regions. This was tested by a "molecular surgical" procedure: HEL was treated with cyanogen bromide, producing a derivative (CB-HEL) with four intact disulfide bonds but strand breaks after the 2 methionine residues at positions 12 and 105 (please see Figure). When CB-HEL, containing the 91–105 determinant cleaved away from the 106–116 determinant, was used to prime (NOD × BALB/c) F1 animals, responses to all 3 determinant envelopes were obtained (17). Thus, this scission within the molecule, effectively separating the two determinants, 91–105 and 106–116, ended the competition and thereby allowed for the enhanced display of the 91–105 region.

The above example emphasizes that competition can occur among different MHC molecules (I-A and I-E) for binding to a stretch of the unfolding antigen, containing distinct determinants. The reverse scenario also exists: different determinants with a range of affinities for a particular class II molecule will compete for binding to the same class II molecule. This competition will be based upon several factors including the position of endopeptidase cleavage sites relative to MHC-binding determinants, the relative MHC affinities of the different determinants, and their location within the molecule. The winning determinant in this competition will be protected from cleavage or removal from its perch within the MHC groove, and therefore will gain access to the surface of the APC. In this "bind first, trim later" scenario, dominant display of a determinant is a direct outcome of the competitive events occurring during processing.

Determinant Hierarchies and the Induction of Tolerance

What happens to the determinants that lose in the competition for MHC binding? Such determinants will likely be destroyed but may receive a second chance at binding if an enzymatic attack frees them from the protected MHC-bound determinant. Thus, binding to the MHC by the winning determinant on the antigen preempts the binding of flanking attached determinants, and thus lowers their functional display. The outcome of these competitive forces is manifested on the surface of the APC as a hierarchy of determinant display (21). In the case of self antigens, only well-displayed determinants will have direct relevance to thymic and peripheral tolerance induction. Thus, T cell repertoires to the cryptic self will remain intact (35–38) and the subdominant self-specific repertoires will only lack their high affinity members (39). T cells specific for dominantly displayed self-determinants will generally be rendered tolerant (36, 37, 40). However, within the dominant determinant envelope certain peptides may nevertheless remain immunogenic. For example, in H-2^d mice 108–116 is the core of the dominant envelope of HEL, 106–122. In HEL-transgenic BALB/c animals, T cell responsiveness to this dominant envelope depends on the level of transgenic HEL expressed. At the lowest level, response to the core 108–116 is lost, but a residual repertoire lacking its highest affinity members to 106–116 remains (41). At higher levels of HEL expression the

106–116 response is completely lost but responses to the longer 108–122 peptide remain (Deng et al., manuscript in preparation). Thus, complete tolerance induction to all the determinants within the envelope is rarely obtained. Since a determinant is usually defined by a set of T cells which binds to an MHC-peptide complex in which the binding residues for the MHC (the agretypic residues) are identical, each T cell within this set can recognize a different group of epitypic residues, which defines its determinant. Thus, peptides of various lengths can contain multiple determinants. Only those which are favored from processing of the intact antigen can be considered "dominant". With regard to the 108–120 determinant of HEL, we would therefore conclude that this peptide contains both the dominant determinant of HEL, 108–116, as well as a second overlapping cryptic one which is not favorably processed from intact HEL or presented. When the peptide 108–120, in the 106–116-tolerant mouse, is used as an immunogen, many T cells are clearly able to respond.

Determinant Spreading

As mentioned, with regards to self protein, an intact T cell repertoire specific for cryptic determinants remains (36, 37). Thus, during an inflammatory response, in which the expression of processing enzymes and MHC molecules is enhanced, the display of these poorly processed and presented determinants can be potentially increased. Since an intact repertoire to these self determinants exists, such an inflammatory event may spark an autoimmune episode. Subsequently, the response may spread by the accumulation of inflammatory events, both intramolecularly and intermolecularly (42, 43).

Retaining Autoreactive T cells to Dominant Determinants of Self-Antigens: Studies of the N-Terminus of Myelin Basic Protein

Another level of complexity arises concerning the dominant determinant in myelin basic protein (MBP) in the $H-2^u$ mouse. Upon immunization with MBP, the amino terminal determinant (acetylated 1–9 or Ac1-9) is the major inducer of T cells, most of which are of rather high affinity. Thus, Ac1-9 is obviously processed efficiently from whole MBP – Why, then, were these high affinity T cells not lost during negative selection? Autoimmune pathology can occur when $H-2^u$ mice are challenged with Ac1–9 or whole MBP. In an effort to learn whether determinant capture might have been involved in protection of these T cells from negative selection, we recently used detector hybridomas to investigate determinant capture within the Golli-MBP protein (genes of the oligodendrocyte lineage-myelin basic protein) (44)(unpublished results). As potential perpetrators of determinant capture, we analyzed the determinants encoded for by the genetic region upstream of the "classical" MBP exons, within what is termed the Golli-MBP gene. The 5' Golli exons are transcribed from their own upstream promoter in frame with the classical MBP exons and truncated products from this gene complex (e.g., BG-21 = Golli1–133; MBP1–57) are found expressed at high levels in the fetal thymus. Importantly, classical MBP has never been detected in the developing thymus. The relatively poor MHC binding affinity of Ac1–9 led us to hypothesize that another, more affine determinant within the context of BG21 might preferentially gain access to the MHC groove, lowering the thymic display of Ac1–9 and thereby preempting tolerance induction to Ac1-9-specific T cells. Therefore, MHC binding studies were conducted on overlapping peptides covering the entire Golli sequence, as well as on the Colli-MBP junctional peptide LDVM1–9 (LDVMASQKRPSQR). Several peptides from the Golli region had the ability to bind significantly to purified I-A^u, LDVM1–9 being the best binder, with a 30-fold better binding affinity than Ac1–9. The lysine residue at position 4 contributes to the poor binding of Acl-9 (45, 46). When this was replaced by each of 10 other residues, but not arginine, the binding of the altered peptide could increase as much as 10,000-fold (met or tyr) (46). Therefore, one of several plausible explanations for the higher binding affinity of LDVM 1–9 relative to Ac1–9 is the existence of an overlapping second determinant with hydrophobic residues at positions –4 (leu) and –1 (met), presumably optimal for binding by I-A^u. The existence of this second determinant would theoretically preempt the binding of the 1–9 sequence of classical MBP, lowering its display and thereby allowing 1–9-reactive cells to escape central tolerance induction. To test this hypothesis we determined the ability of several variant peptides to stimulate LDVM1–9, Ac1–9, and 7–20-specific T cells (Table 1).

Table 1 shows that when the LDVM1–9 determinant ("LDVM") was extended to include 7 additional MBP residues (LDVM1–16), a new dominant determinant was revealed, C-terminal to both the 1–9 and LDVM1–9 registers. Within this 20-mer peptide, the hierarchy of response was 7–16 > LDVM > 1–9. MBP1–9-reactivity was possible only when the key MHC contact residues of both the N-terminal and C-terminal registers of LDVM1–16 were destroyed by replacement with substitute amino acids designed to reduce binding to I-A^u.

Two additional approaches were also employed to demonstrate determinant capture within the Golli-MBP junctional region. In LDVM(1–9)Y4 the 1-9 register could be favored by making the K4Y substitution, which increases the binding of the 1–9-register to I-A^u, achieving a level of parity to the LDVM register. This substitution allowed for recognition of LDVM1–9(Y4) by 1–9-specific T cells, supporting the notion that when flanked by LDVM, the 1–9 register

Table 1. Stimulation of T cell hybridomas specific for:

Peptide	Sequence	LDVM1-9	AC1-9	7-20
Ac1-9	Ac-ASQKRPSQR	–	+++	–
LDVM-(1-9)	LDVMASQKRPSQR	++++	–	–
LDVMR-(2-5)	LDVMRSQKR	–	+++	N.T.
LDVM-(1-9[Y4])	LDVMASQYRPSQR	++++	++++	N.T.
LDVM-(1-16)	LDVMASQKRPSQRSKYLATA	–	–	++++
SDVG-(1-16)	SDVGASQKRPSQRSKYLATA	–	–	++++
LDVM-(1-16[12D,13E])	LDVMASQKRPSQRSKDEATA	++++	–	–
SDVG-(1-16[12D,13E])	SDVGASQKRSQRSKDEATA	–	+++	–

is outcompeted. However, rather than competing for the single optimal binding groove, it was still possible that LDVM actually occupied a different binding site within the MHC groove. To test this, we made use of the principle of molecular mimicry. If the M in LDVM actually competes for occupancy of the same site as the K in Ac1–9, then placement of the key T cell receptor binding residue, arginine, contiguous to the methionine, should allow the recognition by Ac1–9-specific T cells. LDVMR-(2–5) was therefore produced, where methionine serves as an MHC anchor capable of focusing R in just the right position for T cell stimulation. Table 1 shows that this substitution bestowed 1–9-reactivity. These results are consistent with the existence of two registers within LDVM 1–9, an N-terminal dominant register, whose preferential binding to I-A^u prevents the C-terminal 1–9 region from binding to the MHC class II molecule in an appropriate register to permit activation of Ac1–9-specific T cells.

As mentioned earlier, given the preferential binding within LDVM1–16 to the LDVM determinant and the 7–16 determinant, determinant capture should provide double protection for the Ac1–9-specific T cells. Accordingly, this situation represents the prototype of conditions where T cells of high TCR affinity for antigen can be preserved in the self-reactive repertoire, a potentially dangerous threat under the right inflammatory conditions. It is rather common for authors to assume that 1–9 represents an extremely weak determinant (47), and furthermore, that the acetyl group is essential for activity. Our results with the peptide analogue in which both the LDVM and 7–16 registers are inactivated by substitution with inactive amino acids, prove that when freed of its flanking constraints, 1–9 is a potent inducer of specific T cells.

Other experimental systems have also provided evidence for determinant capture, as well as similar types of competition. In one set of experiments, the T cell hierarchy of Golli determinants in the BALB/c mouse was determined. When the binding affinities of overlapping peptides spanning the entire Golli sequence were compared to their immunogenicity, no direct correlation was found. Four peptides were found to bind well to the MHC and of these only two were immunogenic. In fact, Golli p10–24, which was shown to have the strongest affinity for I-A^d, could not induce T cell activation. In contrast, the overlapping, weaker-binding Golli p5–19 was immunogenic (48). Presumably competition by p10–24 for I-A^d preempted the display of p5–19, allowing for 5–19-specific T cells to escape central tolerance induction.

These results parallel findings in the foreign antigen system of Leishmania major. It was shown there that gp63 possessed an array of 3 overlapping determinants 361–375/365–380/and 373–385 (49) of which the central determinant was dominant. In this case, tolerance induced to the long molecule 361–385 led to peripheral tolerance limited to the central dominant determinant, while T cells directed to the flanking determinants had actually been primed by the tolerance-inducing regime. Finally, in the characterization of the T cell determinant structure of mouse lysozyme, ML, it was shown that several ML peptides that bound well to the class II MHC were completely nonimmunogenic when tested in T cell proliferation and cytokine secretion assays, presumably having induced tolerance. In contrast, other ML peptides, known to be "recessive" or "cryptic" in nature, were able to induce proliferative responses (50).

Competition Between T Cells for Their Response to an Antigen

Affinity selection among B cell populations was studied even before the role of T cells was defined. This selection assures the maturation of the highest affinity B cell clones into plasma cells and memory cells. Presumably, driving this selection is the competition of B cells for small residues of antigen (51), making it possible for T cells to drive B cell maturation once this antigen is processed and displayed. In fact, the competitive edge achieved through the early capture of antigen by high affinity variants, and its subsequent presentation in the form of readily processed peptides, provides a target site for ambient T cells. This process thereby simultaneously selects high affinity B cells and high affinity T cells.

Given that there is a broad T cell repertoire directed against any single determinant envelope, we may assume that there is a stochastic distribution of receptor specificities and receptor affinities for the MHC-Ag ligand. Furthermore, other surface molecules play a role in the efficiency of constituting the MHC- T cell synapse. An assumption that appears to be borne out in the few experiments actually performed to examine the topic, is that the dominant T cell has a high affinity for antigen.

Although competition for antigen among T cells has been demonstrated in vitro, evidence for this phenomenon in vivo is under scrutiny. A few recent publications have demonstrated that T cells with high affinity TCRs become rapidly dominant and are eventually selected for memory responses (52, 53). In particular, the role of antigen-APC in determining the fate of T cell competition and the eventual selection of high affinity TCRs has been investigated. Studies by Kedl et al. (54) present data that CD8[+] T cells can compete with each other during responses to antigen in vivo. In these studies using a transgenic TCR system they show that T cell-APC interactions determine the fate of T cell selection. Their studies further show that successful competition between T cells does not require that the T cells respond to the same determinant, nor does it involve the killing of the APC. They suggest that the competition between CD8[+] T cells in gaining access to MHC-linked antigen may be due to limited availability for soluble growth factors or MHC/costimulatory molecules on the APC for the T cells. Another set of studies by Smith et al (55) to investigate the competition between CD4[+] T cells has employed CFSE labeled transgenic TCR T cells to allow direct visualization of effects of in vivo competition at the level of individual responder cells. These studies suggest that the quality of the immune response is independent of the initial precursor frequency of responders. They further show that regardless of wide variations in affinities and frequencies of the TCRs selected, the competition for antigen allows the activation of the highest affinity T cells; also, the amount of available antigen serves to determine the final size of the effector T cell response. In contrast to the studies by Kedl, the studies by Smith et al. suggest that competition is restricted to T cells of the same specificity, suggesting that T cells compete for an antigen-MHC complex rather than for antigen non-specific factors.

Memory Resides in T Cell Clones of Intermediate Affinty

Thus, in certain circumstances, the high affinity clone appears to prevail and subsequently dominate the immune response: however, there are notable exceptions. During the course of EAE, we have seen that the initiating dominant MBP Ac1–9-specific clone, whose pathogenic attributes have led us to call it a "driver clone", is purged from the repertoire, leaving behind a residual repertoire of possible lower affinity/Th2 cells and a recovered mouse resistant to disease reinduction (56). Similarly, when tolerance is induced to the dominant determinant of HEL, the dominant, high affinity clone is lost from the repertoire, leaving Th2 clones to dominate the "tolerant" response (40).

It is of particular interest that dominant clones in these studies are public (i.e. common to all individual animals), while the residual, lower affinity clones are private (i.e. differ from one animal to the next). What attributes lead to a particular clone being public? A number of studies suggest that this selection is independent of precursor frequency (55,57). Also, as described above, affinity presumably plays a role.

Fasso et al. have seen that intermediate affinity clones were selected to lead the memory response to sperm whale myoglobin (SWM) (58). This would be expected from a model in which high affinity clones might be the first to be activated, but then become selected against (e.g. through activation-induced-cell-death), leaving behind sets of lower affinity clones. Alternatively, it is worth mentioning that affinity is the combined contribution of the on-rate and the off-rate. Optimal signaling will obviously benefit from a fast on-rate, but it has been suggested that a relatively fast off-rate may enhance signaling through "serial triggering" (59). Thus, we may often see intermediate affinity clones winning the competition by being able to disengage and be subsequently triggered by a new synaptic interaction.

Degeneracy and Plasticity of the T Cell Receptor

In the context of tissue inflammation or infection with a microorganism, one can expect many determinants to be displayed on the surface of an APC. Despite the limits imposed by antigen processing and T cell availability, a wide variety of determinants from a plethora of antigens will be displayed in any given environment (11, 31, 60, 61) (aside from the artificial situation where a single antigen is used for immunization). Degeneracy of T cell receptor recognition seems to be a general rule, an evolutionary consequence of the limited number of TCR contact sites and of plasticity in the CDR3 region (62). For example, in the MBP-specific response of the B10.PL mouse, the public set of T cells have the CDR3 sequence DAGGGY (56, 63). The stretch of glycines appears to provide extensive flexibility and thereby promote repertoire degeneracy. It is estimated that, for CD4+ T cells, a single T cell receptor can recognize as many as 10^6 different peptides (64–66). Since optimal stimulation of T cells relates to a high density of the ligand matrix on the surface of the APC, those T cells which have the most degenerate TCRs and recognize multiple determinants in a given antigenic environment may be highly selected on this basis. This concept was demonstrated by Schumacher and colleagues using two variants of viral peptides (67). Although cross-reactive T cells were very rare in the original T cell pool responding to the first peptide, there was a selective expansion of the cross-reactive pool, such that these cells dominated the secondary response when the variant peptide was used to rechallenge. Extending these results to a multi-determinant situation, one can envision that a clonal hierarchy is established, within which the most dominant clone may be that one which recognizes multiple determinants from the environment. **The CD4+ T cell may thus act as a pattern recognizer, achieving specificity not at the single determinant level, but at the level of the determinant milieu as a whole.**

In summary, the final readout of immunization is revealed in the T and B cell populations which are engaged, the final result being the outcome of a series of competitions. With the B cell, the most highly affine member will bind the determinant on the native antigen, leading to the most rapid production of a signalling peptide which through T cell recognition, then drives the favored B cell to mature. T cells of the highest affinity for the initially displayed determinant will win a T cell competition, and the result will be a dual selection of the most appropriate T and B cells. Mutations in the affinity of the B cell receptor for the native antigen will lead to the most rapid display of the dominant determinant. If we now consider the APC population as a whole, wandering T cells may encounter different dominant determinants from the same antigen displayed on different APC. (In most cases, well-expressed determinants seem to be dominantly expressed by all APC, but this is a poorly studied area). The crucial molecules influencing CD4 T cell immunodominance are the endopeptidases which make the first nick in tightly folded antigenic molecules, rendering them available for binding to MHC class II molecules. The most readily available determinant near the peptide scission site will usually become the dominant determinant. T cells with high avidity receptors, and efficient costimulatory receptors will also compete for selection. Interestingly, in all animals of a particular strain, certain public T cells have the "right stuff" to be selected consistently, suggesting that there may not be as much variability in the whole population of T cells specific for certain determinants.

What is clear from these studies is that (a) competition occurs at the level of B cell receptors, T cell receptors, and MHC grooves (b) immunodominance results from this intertwined series of selections (c) the initially selected T cells, owing to regulation or activation induced cell death, may not be the T cells which comprise the memory response or which remain to protect the individual from recurrent infections. The notion of "survival of the fittest" may evolve to "survival of the apparently not-so-fit".

Acknowledgments

This work was supported by grants from the National Multiple Sclerosis Society and the N.I.H. awarded to E.E.S. Emanual Maverakis is an HHMI medical student fellow. Jonathan Beech and Peter van den Elzen are postdoctoral fellows of the NMSS. This is manuscript number 417 of the La Jolla Institute for Allergy and Immunology.

References

1. Gell PGH, Benacerraf B (1959) Studies on hypersensitivity .2. Delayed Hypersensitivity To Denatured Proteins In Guinea Pigs. Immunology 2:64
2. Sette A, Adorini L, Colon SM, Buus S, Grey HM (1989) Capacity of intact proteins to bind to MHC class II molecules. J Immunol 143:1265
3. Bjorkman PJ, Saper MA,. Samraoui B, Bennett WS, Strominger JL, Wiley DC (1987) Structure of the human class I histocompatibility antigen, HLA-A2. Nature 329:506
4. Madden DR, Gorga JC, Strominger JL, Wiley DC (1991) The structure of HLA-B27 reveals nonamer self-peptides bound in an extended conformation. Nature 353:321
5. Fremont DH, Matsumura M, Stura EA, Peterson PA, Wilson IA (1992) Crystal structures of two viral peptides in complex with murine MHC class 1 H-2Kb [see comments]. Science 257:919
6. Stern LJ, Brown JH, Jardetzky TS, Gorga JC, Urban RG, Strominger JL, Wiley DC (1994) Crystal structure of the human class II MHC protein HLA-DR1 complexed with an influenza virus peptide. Nature 368:215
7. Degano M, Garcia KC, Apostolopoulos V, Rudolph MG, Teyton L, Wilson A (2000) A functional hot spot for antigen recognition in a superagonist TCR/MHC complex. Immunity 12:251
8. Hennecke J, Carfi A, Wiley DC (2000) Structure of a covalently stabilized complex of a human alphabeta T-cell receptor, influenza HA peptide and MHC class II molecule, HLA-DR1. Embo J 19:5611
9. Baker MB, Gagnon JS, Biddison EW, Wiley DC (2000) Conversion of a T cell antagonist into an agonist by repairing a defect in the TCR/peptide/MHC interface: implications for TCR signaling. Immunity 13:475
10. Reinherz EL, Tan K, Tang L, Kern P, Liu J, Xiong Y, Hussey RE, Smolyar A, Hare B, Zhang R, Joachimiak A, Chang HC, Wagner G, Wang J (1999) The crystal structure of a T cell receptor in complex with peptide and MHC class II. Science 286:1913
11. Rudensky A, Preston-Hurlburt P, Hong SC, Barlow A, Janeway CA Jr (1991) Sequence analysis of peptides bound to MHC class II molecules [see comments]. Nature 353:622
12. Sette A, Adorini L, Colon SM, Buus S, Grey HM (1989) Capacity of intact proteins to bind to MHC class II molecules. J Immunol 143:1265
13. Castellino F, Zappacosta F, Coligan JE, Germain RN (1998) Large protein fragments as substrates for endocytic antigen capture by MHC class II molecules. J Immunol 161:4048
14. Lee P, Matsueda GR, Allen PM (1988) T cell recognition of fibrinogen. A determinant on the A alpha-chain does not require processing. J Immunol 140:1063

15. Donermeyer DL, Allen PM (1989) Binding to Ia protects an immunogenic peptide from proteolytic degradation. J Immunol 142:1063

16. Mouritsen S, Meldal M, Werdelin O, Hansen AS, Buus S (1992) MHC molecules protect T cell epitopes against proteolytic destruction. J Immunol 149:1987

17. Deng H, Apple R, Clare-Salzler M, Trembleau S, Mathis D, Adorini L, Sercarz E (1993) Determinant capture as a possible mechanism of protection afforded by major histocompatibility complex class II molecules in autoimmune disease. J Exp Med 178:1675

18. Manoury BE, Hewitt W, Morrice N, Dando PM, Barrett AJ, Watts C (1998) An asparaginyl endopeptidase processes a microbial antigen for class II MHC presentation. Nature 396:695

19. Schneider SC, Ohmen J, Fosdick L, Gladstone B, Guo J, Ametani A, Sercarz EE, Deng H (2000) Cutting edge: introduction of an endopeptidase cleavage motif into a determinant flanking region of hen egg lysozyme results in enhanced T cell determinant display. J Immunol 165:20

20. Berzofsky JA, Richman LK, Killion DJ (1979) Distinct H-2-linked Ir genes control both antibody and T cell responses to different determinants on the same antigen, myoglobin. Proc Natl Acad Sci USA 76:4046

21. Katz ME, Maizels RM, Wieker L, Miller A, Sercarz EE (1982) Immunological focusing by the mouse major histocompatibility complex: mouse strains confronted with distantly related lysozymes confine their attention to very few epitopes. Eur J Immunol 12:535

22. Barcinski MA, Rosenthal AS (1977) Immune response gene control of determinant selection. I. Intramolecular mapping of the immunogenic sites on insulin recognized by guinea pig T and B cells. J Exp Med 145:726

23. Cohen IR, Talmon J (1980) H-2 genetic control of the response of T lymphocytes to insulins. Priming of nonresponder mice by forbidden variants of specific antigenic determinants. Eur J Immunol 10:284

24. Roy S, Scherer MT, Briner TJ, Smith JA, Gefter ML (1989) Murine MHC polymorphism and T cell specificities. Science 244:572

25. Nanda NK, Apple R, Sercarz E (1991) Limitations in plasticity of the T-cell receptor repertoire. Proc Natl Acad Sci USA 88:9503

26. Moudgil KD, Grewal IS, Jensen PE, Sercarz EE (1996) Unresponsiveness to a self-peptide of mouse lysozyme owing to hindrance of T cell receptor-major histocompatibility complex/peptide interaction caused by flanking epitopic residues. J Exp Med 183:535

27. Sercarz EE, Lehmann PV, Ametani A, Benichou G, Miller A, Moudgil K (1993) Dominance and crypticity of T cell antigenic determinants. Annu Rev Immunol 11:729

28. Grewal IS, Moudgil KD, Sercarz EE (1995) Hindrance of binding to class II major histocompatibility complex molecules by a single amino acid residue contiguous to a determinant leads to crypticity of the determinant as well as lack of response to the protein antigen. Proc Natl Acad Sci USA 92:1779

29. Moudgil KD, Sercarz EE, Grewal IS (1998) Modulation of the immunogenicity of antigenic determinants by their flanking residues. Immunol Today 19:217

30. Viner NJ, Nelson CA, Unanue ER (1995) Identification of a major I-Ek-restricted determinant of hen egg lysozyme: limitations of lymph node proliferation studies in defining immunodominance and crypticity. Proc Natl Acad Sci USA 92:2214

31. Chicz RM, Urban RG, Lane WS, Gorga JC, Stern LJ, Vignali DA, Strominger JL (1992) Predominant naturally processed peptides bound to HLA-DR1 are derived from MHC-related molecules and are heterogeneous in size. Nature 358:764

32. Drakesmith H, O'Neil D, Schneider SC, Binks M, Medd P, Sercarz E, Beverley P, Cham B (1998) In vivo priming of T cells against cryptic determinants by dendritic cells exposed to interleukin 6 and native antigen. Proc Natl Acad Sci USA 95:14903

33. Schneider SC, Ohmen J, Fosdick L, Gladstone B, Guo J, Ametani A, Sercarz EE, Deng H (2000) Cutting edge: introduction of an endopeptidase cleavage motif into a determinant flanking region of hen egg lysozyme results in enhanced T cell determinant display. J Immunol 165:20

34. Gammon G, Geysen HM, Apple RJ, Pickett E, Palmer M, Ametani A, Sercarz EE (1991) T cell determinant structure: cores and determinant envelopes in three mouse major histocompatibility complex haplotypes. J Exp Med 173:609

35. Ria F, Chan BM, Scherer MT, Smith JA, Gefter ML (1990) Immunological activity of covalently linked T-cell epitopes. Nature 343:381

36. Gammon G, Sercarz E (1989) How some T cells escape tolerance induction. Nature 342:183

37. Cibotti R, Kanellopoulos JM, Cabaniols JP, Halle-Panenko O, Kosmatopoulos K, Sercarz E, Kourilsky P (1992) Tolerance to a self-protein involves its immunodominant but does not involve its subdominant determinants. Proc Natl Acad Sci USA 89:416

38. Wilson SS, Elzen van den P, Maverakis E, Beech JT, Braciak TA, Kumar V, Sercarz EE (2000) Residual public repertoires to self. J Neuroimmunol 107:233

39. Gapin L, Cabaniols JP, Cibotti R, Ojcius DM, Kourilsky P, Kanellopoulos JM (1997) Determinant selection for T-cell tolerance in HEL-transgenic mice: dissociation between immunogenicity and tolerogenicity. Cell Immunol 177:77

40. Maverakis E, Beech JT, Wilson SS, Quinn A, Pedersen B, Sercarz EE (2000) T cell receptor complementarity determining region 3 length analysis reveals the absence of a characteristic public T cell repertoire in neonatal tolerance. The response in the "tolerant" mouse within the residual repertoire is quantitatively similar but qualitatively different. J Exp Med 191:695

41. Cibotti R, Cabaniols JP, Pannetier C, Delarbre C, Vergnon I, Kanellopoulos JM, Kourilsky P (1994) Public and private V beta T cell receptor repertoires against hen egg white lysozyme (HEL) in nontransgenic versus HEL transgenic mice. J Exp Med 180:861

42. Lehmann PV, Forsthuber T, Miller A, Sercarz EE (1992) Spreading of T-cell autoimmunity to cryptic determinants of an autoantigen. Nature 358:155

43. McRae BL, Vanderlugt CL, Dal Canto MC, Miller SD (1995) Functional evidence for epitope spreading in the relapsing pathology of experimental autoimmune encephalomyelitis. J Exp Med 182:75

44. Maverakis E, Stevens DB, Brossay L, Mendoza R, Macias L, Skinner E, Sette A, Campagnoni A, Sercarz E (1996) Determinant capture by flanking Golli determinant protects dominant MBP N-terminal-specific T cells from negative selection. FASEB Journal 10:1226

45. Wraith DC, Smilek DE, Mitchell DJ, Steinman L, McDevitt HO (1989) Antigen recognition in autoimmune encephalomyelitis and the potential for peptide-mediated immunotherapy. Cell 59:247

46. Kumar V, Bhardwaj V, Soares L, Alexander J, Sette A, Sercarz E (1995) Major histocompatibility complex binding affinity of an antigenic determinant is crucial for the differential secretion of interleukin 4/5 or interferon gamma by T cells. Proc Natl Acad Sci USA 92:9510

47. Liu GY, Fairchild PJ, Smith RM, Prowle JR, Kioussis D, Wraith DC (1995) Low avidity recognition of self-antigen by T cells permits escape from central tolerance. Immunity 3:407

48. Maverakis E, Mendoza R, Southwood S, Raja-Gabaglia C, Abromson-Leeman S, Campagnoni AT, Sette A, Sercarz EE (2000) Immunogenicity of self antigens is unrelated to MHC-binding affinity: T-cell determinant structure of golli-MBP in the BALB/c mouse [In Process Citation]. J Autoimmun 15:315

49. Soares LR, Serearz EE, Miller A (1994) Vaccination of the Leishmania major susceptible BALB/c mouse. I. The precise selection of peptide determinant influences CD4+ T cell subset expression. Int Immunol 6:785

50. Moudgil KD, Southwood S, Ametani A, Kim K, Sette A, Sercarz EE (1999) The self-directed T cell repertoire against mouse lysozyme reflects the influence of the hierarchy of its own determinants and can be engaged by a foreign lysozyme. J Immunol 163:4232

51. Manser T, Parhami-Seren B, Margolies MN, Gefter ML (1987) Somatically mutated forms of a major anti-p-azophenylarsonate antibody variable region with drastically reduced affinity for p-azophenylarsonate. By-products of an antigen-driven immune response? J Exp Med 166:1456

52. Savage PA, Boniface JJ, Davis MM (1999) A kinetic basis for T cell receptor repertoire selection during an immune response. Immunity 10:485

53. McHeyzer-Williams LJ, Panus JF, Mikszta JA, McHeyzer-Williams MG (1999) Evolution of antigen-specific T cell receptors in vivo: preimmune and antigen-driven selection of preferred complementarity-determining region 3 (CDR3) motifs. J Exp Med 189:1823

54. Kedl RM, Rees WA, Hildeman DA, Schaefer B, Mitchell T, Kappler J, Marrack P (2000) T cells compete for access to antigen-bearing antigen-presenting cells. J Exp Med 192:1105

55. Smith AL, Wikstrom ME, Fazekas de St Groth B (2000) Visualizing T cell Competition for Peptide/MHC Complexes. A Specific Mechanism to Minimize the Effect of Precursor Frequency. Immunity 13:783

56. van den Elzen P, Maverakis E, Kumar V, Wilson S, Sercarz E (2001) A repertoire shift is a key feature in recovery from autoimmunity: loss of driver T cells and maintenance of a benign repertoire. submitted

57. Radu CG, Anderton SM, Firan M, Wraith DC, Ward ES (2000) Detection of autoreactive T cells in H-2u mice using peptide-MHC multimers. Int Immunol 12:1553

58. Fasso M, Anandasabapathy N, Crawford F, Kappler J, Fathman CG, Ridgway WM (2000) T cell receptor (TCR)-mediated repertoire selection and loss of TCR vbeta diversity during the initiation of a CD4(+) T cell response in vivo. J Exp Med 192:1719

59. Valitutti S, Muller S, Cella M, Padovan E, and Lanzavecchia A (1995) Serial triggering of many T-cell receptors by a few peptide-MHC complexes. Nature 375:148

60. Chicz RM, Urban RG, Gorga JC, Vignali DA, Lane WS, Strominger JL (1993) Specificity and promiscuity among naturally processed peptides bound to HLA-DR alleles. J Exp Med 178:27

61. Hunt DF, Michel H, Dickinson TA, Shabanowitz J, Cox AL, Sakaguchi K, Appella E, Grey HM, Sette A (1992) Peptides presented to the immune system by the murine class II major histocompatibility complex molecule I-Ad. Science 256:1817

62. Hare BJ, Wyss DF, Osburne MS, Kern PS, Reinherz EL, Wagner F (1999) Structure, specificity and CDR mobility of a class II restricted single-chain T-cell receptor. Nat Struct Biol 6:574

63. Urban JL, Kumar V, Kono DH, Gomez C, Horvath SJ, Clayton J, Ando DG, Sercarz EE, Hood L (1988) Restricted use of T cell receptor V genes in murine autoimmune encephalomyelitis raises possibilities for antibody therapy. Cell 54:577

64. Wilson DB, Pinilla C, Wilson DH, Schroder K, Boggiano C, Judkowski V, Kaye J, Hemmer B, Martin R, Houghten RA (1999) Immunogenicity. I. Use of peptide libraries to identify epitopes that activate clonotypic CD4+ T cells and induce T cell responses to native peptide ligands. J Immunol 163:6424

65. Mason D (1998) A very high level of crossreactivity is an essential feature of the T-cell receptor [see comments]. Immunol Today 19:395

66. Maverakis E, Elzen van den P, Sercarz EE (2001) Self-reactive T cells and Degeneracy of T cell Recognition: evolving concepts --from sequence homology to shape mimicry and TCR flexibility. Journal of Autoimmunity 16

67. Haanen JB, Wolkers MC, Kruisbeek AM, Schumacher TN (1999) Selective expansion of cross-reactive CD8(+) memory T cells by viral variants. J Exp Med 190:1319

Using Monoclonal Antibodies and Site Directed Mutagenesis to Map the Epitopes of the Blood Group Rh D Antigen

M. Scott[1], D. Voak[2], W. Liu[1,3], J.W. Jones[1,4,] and N.D. Avent[1,5]

Brief History of the Discovery of the Rh Blood Group System

In 1939 Levine & Stetson [1] investigated a case of a mother, delivered of a stillborn child, having a haemolytic transfusion reaction after being given her husband's blood. Her serum agglutinated her husband's red cells and those of 80 % of ABO compatible donors. They showed that this new antigen, to which they did not assign a name, was different to the then known blood groups ABO, MN and P. They hypothesised that the mother had been immunised to produce antibody by an antigen of paternal origin present in the foetus, and that the haemolytic transfusion reaction was due to this antibody reacting with the same antigen on her husband's red cells.

In 1940 Landsteiner & Wiener [2] injected rhesus monkey red cells into rabbits. The rabbit serum agglutinated rhesus monkey red cells, and also the red cells from 85 % of white residents in New York. They called the antibody anti-Rh. Studies of 60 families showed that positivity with the antiserum was inherited as a dominant allele [3]. Wiener & Peters [4] identified antibodies of apparently the same specificity in patients who had transfusion reactions after receiving ABO incompatible blood. In 1941 studies indicated that the antibody described by Levine & Stetson in 1939 had the same specificity as the anti-Rh serum [5].

However, in 1942 studies demonstrated that there were differences between animal and human anti-Rh [6] – red cells from all newborn babies reacted with animal anti-Rh, whereas only 85 % reacted with human anti-Rh. Twenty years later it was confirmed that the human and animal anti-Rh antibodies did not

[1] Bristol Institute for Transfusion Sciences, Bristol, UK
[2] National Blood Service, Cambridge, UK
[3] Dept of Haematology, Hong Kong University, Hong Kong
[4] National Blood Service, Liverpool, UK
[5] University of the West of England, Bristol, UK

react with the same antigen [7]. The nomenclature of "Rh" for the antigens recognised by the human "anti-Rh" antibodies had by this time been used in numerous publications, and was in common usage. Levine [7] therefore proposed that the human antigen and antibodies should carry on being called Rh, but that the specificity defined by the animal sera should be renamed LW, in honour of Landsteiner and Wiener. Many sources accredit the discovery of the Rh blood groups to Landsteiner and Wiener – in fact they discovered the LW blood group system, not Rh!

By 1943 Wiener [8] had demonstrated 6 alleles within the Rh system. Later studies confirmed the existence of 5 antigens within the Rh system, four of which formed antithetical pairs. The three independent antigens were called C, D and E, with the antithetical antigen of C being termed c and that of E being termed e. Levine and colleagues in several studies [5, 9, 10] demonstrated that Rh D incompatibility between mother and foetus was the major cause of haemolytic disease of the newborn (HDN). The finding in 1960 that Rh D negative women can be treated with prophylactic anti-D to prevent HDN is one of the great successes of modern medicine. Various later studies showed that, depending on the population group studied, 3–25 % of the population lack the Rh D antigen. Rh D negative individuals readily make anti-D if challenged with Rh D positive blood – 80 % of cases will make anti-D if they receive a unit of Rh D positive blood, and 16 % of Rh D negative pregnant women carrying Rh D positive foetuses will make anti-D, unless suitable prophylactic anti-D is given [11]. Rh D is thus of critical importance in blood transfusion.

Development of the Hypothesis that the Rh D Antigen is a Mosaic of Many Epitopes

Qualitative variants of Rh D were first discovered when rare D-positive individuals were found to have made allo-anti-D in response to blood transfusion with Rh D positive blood [12]. Their red cells were considered to lack "part" of the normal D antigen, such that they had made anti-D to the missing "part" on challenge with the whole D antigen. Thus they were called "partial" D. Blood samples with partial D antigens were studied by Wiener, Unger and their colleagues [13] – they named the components of the Rh D antigen Rh^A, Rh^B, Rh^C and Rh^D. In 1962, Tippett and Sanger [14] studied the interactions of cells and serum from D positive people who had anti-D in their serum. They observed a limited number of reaction patterns and divided samples with partial D antigens into six categories. The specificity of the anti-D antibodies made by members of the same category was not identical but, by definition, cells and sera of members of the same category were mutually compatible.

Category I was an exception. This was a heterogeneous collection of D-positive people reported to have made allo-anti-D, but their antibody was no longer active when they were retested in 1962. Category I was thus declared obsolete.

Subsequently, most categories were sub-divided and another category, category VII, was added to accommodate D-positive Tar+ (RH:1,40) people who had made anti-D. The pattern of interactions between the categories and subcategories is complex (Table 1). Recently two more partial D phenotypes have been identified. These were called DFR [15] and DBT [16], as it was not possible to give them category numbers because the cross-testing required to establish a new category was not possible. More partial D phenotypes have since been described due to their discrepant reactions with monoclonal antibody reagents – again these have not been added to the category system – see below. The phenotype $R_0^{Har}r$ was also not defined with the category system, as the cells gave discrepant reactions with anti-D from category individuals.

Table 1. Interactions of cells and anti-D in sera of people with partial D antigens who have made anti-D

Cells	Anti-D From:							
	II	IIIa	IIIc	IVa	IVb	Va	Vb	VI
II	0	+	+	+	w	+	+	+
IIIa	+	0	0	+	+	+	+	+
IIIb	+	0	0	+	+	w	+	+
IIIc	+	0	0	+	+	+	+	+
IVa	0	w	0	0	0	+	+	+
IVb	0	w	w	0	0	0	+	*
Va	+	0	0	+	+	0	w	*
VI	0	0	0	*	*	0	0	0
VII	+	*	*	+	+	*	+	+
DFR	+	0	*	+	+	0	0	0
DBT	0	nt	w	0	0	*	+	*

* + with some sera, 0 with other sera.
w = weak reaction
nt = not tested.

Further Work on Rh D Epitopes Using Monoclonal Antibodies

The successful production of a large number of different human monoclonal anti-D antibodies has provided newer tools for the investigation of partial D phenotypes. Indeed, the widespread use of two monoclonal Rh D typing reagents side-by-side in routine practice has resulted in the identification of further partial D individuals who have not yet necessarily made allo-anti-D.

Different patterns of reaction were observed when monoclonal anti-D were tested with partial D category red cells – these were presumed to represent different epitopes – that is different specific binding sites for the antibodies. Studies by Dr. Tippett's group have indicated that at least nine epitopes are suggested by the pattern of reactivity of MAbs with D category cells (17). Table 2 shows the reaction patterns of examples of monoclonal anti-D's with rare types of red cells from D categories (D positive with anti-D in their serum), D variants (D positive with missing epitopes but no anti-D) and with weak D types. New

Table 2. Reactivity of Examples of IgM Monoclonal anti-D with D category, variant and weak D cells

cell	RUM-1	BS226	MAD-2	HAM-A	B10
II	+	+	+	+	–
III	+	+	+	+	+
IVa	+	+	+	+	–
IVb	+	+	+	+	–
Va	+	+	+/–	–	+
VI	–	–	–	–	+
VII	+	+	+	+	+
DFR	+	–	–	–	–
DHMi	+	+	+	–	–
DHMii	+	+	+	–	+
Rh:32	+	+	–	–	–
R_0^{Har}	+	+	–	–	–
weak D*	6	4	2	1	1

* Average reaction grade with weak D, on a scale 0 to 6.

D variants are being discovered with the increased routine use of monoclonal anti-D reagents, and many of these do not fit with the reaction patterns of known D categories or variants (18). DHMi, DHMii, DNU, DHR and DMH are some examples.

It is important to note that some reaction patterns are concentration and technique dependent. For example, at high concentrations MAD-2 will react with D^{Va} category cells; at lower concentrations it will not. This is in contrast to other MAbs, such as RUM-1, that react with D^{Va} cells over a range of concentrations and others, such as HAM-A, that do not react with D^{Va} at even high concentrations of MAb. Some MAbs only react with a particular variant red cell after the cell has been enzyme treated. In contrast, the reactivity of one MAb (MS26) with certain category and variant cells is abolished after enzyme treatment of the cells.

Studies by the International Council for Standards in Haematology/International Society for Blood Transfusion working party on blood grouping reagents (reported at the Amsterdam ISBT meeting, July 1994) examined the reaction patterns of 38 monoclonal anti-D's with 80 category and variant red cells, untreated and enzyme treated. The results suggested that there may be 20 or more different patterns of reactivity of MAb anti-D with variant cells. The ISBT 3rd Monoclonal Workshop reported in Nantes, 1996, examined the reaction patterns of 168 monoclonal antibodies with 375 variant red cell samples (untreated and enzyme treated) in 43 labs (19). Both these studies were multi-centre evaluations using standard methods and evaluation of each antibody at three different dilutions. The latter study concluded that patterns observed with enzyme treated red cells were too variable between labs to be used for classification. From the results of this study, 24 Rh D epitopes have been defined by clusters of monoclonal antibodies (Table 3) [19]. A fourth ISBT Monoclonal workshop is currently underway, to be reported in Paris in July 2001. Further panels of monoclonal anti-D are being tested with D variant red cells in laboratories around the world.

Selection of Epitope Specific Monoclonal Antibodies as Blood Grouping Reagent

To date, not one monoclonal anti-D has been produced that will react with all types of variants of the D antigen. There has therefore been much debate as to which monoclonal antibodies are suitable as routine blood grouping reagents.

For donor typing it is important to type all presentations of Rh D that could cause immunisation in a D negative individual as D positive. Use of a single monoclonal anti-D is therefore not acceptable. A single polyclonal anti-D can

Table 3. Division of MAbs from the 3rd monoclonal workshop into Reaction Patterns

a) those fitting previously decribed patterns

1–9	1–31	Nantes	II	IIIa	IIIb	IIIc	IVa	IVb	Va	VI	VII	DFR	DBT	Ro^{Har}	HMi
1	1	82, 123	+	+	+	+	–	–	–	++	–	–	+	–	–
1	2	79, 83	+	+	+	+	–	–	–	–	+	–	–	–	+
2	3	44, 51	+	+	+	+	–	–	+	–	+	+	–	–	+
3	5	43, 49, 75, 106, 131, 179	+	+	+	+	–	–	+	+	+	+	–	–	+
4	6	45	–	+	+	+	+	–	+	+	+	+	–	–	+
5	7	42, 116	+	+	+	+	+	+	–	–	+	+	–	+	+
5	8	56, 59, 114	+	+	+	+	+	+	–	–	+	+	–	–	+
5	10	41, 52, 70, 88, 89, 109, 110, 130	+	+	+	+	+	+	–	–	+	–	–	–	+
5	11	48, 69	+	+	+	+	+	+	–	–	+	–	–	–	–
6/7	12	35, 46, 102, 103, 113, 125, 128	+	+	+	+	+	+	+	–	+	+	+	+	+
6/7	13	29, 36, 47, 90, 93, 106	+	+	+	+	+	+	+	–	+	+	+	–	+
6/7	14	58	+	+	+	+	+	+	+	–	+	+	–	+	+
6/7	15	31, 32, 71, 80, 95, 97, 108	+	+	+	+	+	+	+	–	+	+	–	–	+
6/7	16	81	+	+	+	+	+	+	+	–	+	+	–	–	+
6/7	17	28, 34, 37, 39, 98, 99, 111, 115, 134	+	+	+	+	+	+	+	–	+	–	+	+	+
6/7	18	30, 84, 85, 86, 87, 100, 119, 126	+	+	+	+	+	+	+	–	+	–	+	–	+
6/7	21	33, 94, 104	+	+	+	+	+	+	+	–	+	–	–	–	+
8	22	74, 78	+	+	+	+	+	+	+	–	–	–	+	–	–
9	23	77, 96, 101, 112, 118, 120, 121, 127	–	+	+	+	–	–	+	+	+	+	–	–	+

b) new patterns

1–9	1–31	Nantes	II	IIIa	IIIb	IIIc	IVa	IVb	Va	VI	VII	DFR	DBT	R$_o$^{Har}	HMi
	31	54, 57, 62	+	+	+	+	+	–	–	–	–	–	–	–	–
	32	38	+	+	+	+	+	+	+	–	+	–	+	–	–
	33	50	+	+	+	+	+	–	+	–	+	+	–	–	–
	34	60	+	+	+	+	+	–	+	–	+	+	–	–	+
	35	53, 55, 72, 76	+	+	+	+	+	–	+	+	+	+	–	–	+
	36	73, 68, 124, 117, 180	+	+	+	+	+	+	+	+	+	+	+	–	+

be used if it has been shown to adequately detect weak D and D variants including category VI. The most common policy is to use one saline monoclonal anti-D that gives strong reactivity with normal D phenotypes, but does not react with D^{VI}, alongside a polyclonal or other monoclonal reagent that has been specifically selected for detection of D^{VI}.

For patient and pregnant woman typing, it is theoretically best if all D variant phenotype individuals are typed as D negative, as they will then safely be given D negative blood and not immunised against the epitopes of the D antigen that they lack.

Partial D pregnant women will also then be given prophylactic anti-D to prevent immunisation by fetal Rh D antigen. However, this approach is not practical, as a large panel of monoclonal anti-D would have to be tested to identify every type of D variant. D^{VI} individuals lack much of the normal D antigen, and readily make potent anti-D when transfused with D positive blood. D^{VI} mothers have been shown to make anti-D that causes clinically severe haemolytic disease of the newborn. Reagents used for routine patient and pregnant woman typing should therefore not detect D^{VI}.

Biochemistry of Rh

In 1982, Moore et al [20] showed that anti-D immunoprecipitated a protein of 30,000 molecular weight from red cells. Immunoprecipitation with monoclonal anti-c or anti-E yielded a protein with a molecular weight 2000 higher than the protein immunoprecipitated by anti-D [21]. One and two-dimensional peptide maps of the immunoprecipitated proteins confirmed that the Rh D and CcEe antigens are expressed on similar but distinct polypeptides [22]. Neither polypeptide is glycosylated. In addition to the Rh D and Rh CE polypeptides, a larger polypeptide of approximately 50,000 molecular weight co-precipitated. This polypeptide was shown to be a glycoprotein, known as the Rh associated glycoprotein. The Rh polypeptides and the Rh associated glycoprotein exist as non-covalently bound complexes in the native red cell membrane.

Molecular Biology of Rh D

In 1990 the gene corresponding to the CcEe Rh protein was cloned [23, 24]. In 1992 the gene corresponding to the D Rh protein was cloned [25]. The nucleotide sequences of both genes predicted polypeptides with 417 amino acid polypeptides, with the Rh D sequence differing from the Rh CcEe sequence in only 36 amino acids. In 1991, Colin et al showed that RHCE and RHD genes are present in all Rh D positive individuals, whereas only *RHCE* is present in Rh D negative individuals [26]. Rh D negative individuals appear to completely lack the *RHD* gene, and thus their red cells contain no Rh D polypeptide. This explains why Rh D negative individuals so readily make anti-D, and why the antibody response consists of antibodies with different fine epitope specificities – the immune response is being mounted to a whole foreign protein, which has many epitopes.

Both *RH* genes are organised into 10 exons [27]. Hydropathy plots of the predicted primary amino acid sequence indicate a very similar membrane organisation for the two Rh proteins, predicting 12 transmembrane domains, 6 extracellular loops and cytoplasmic N and C termini. Only nine of the Rh D specific residues are predicted to be exposed at the extracellular surface of the red cell: 1 in extracellular loop 2, 3 in extracellular loop 3, 2 in extracellular loop 4 and 3 in extracellular loop 6. This model is shown in Figure 1.

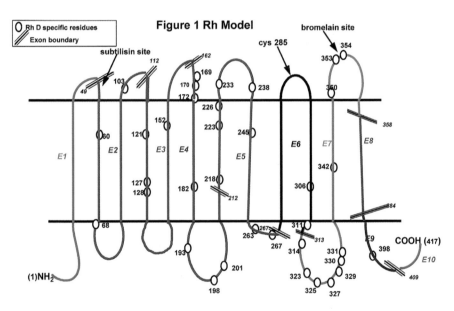

Fig. 1. Model of the Rh polypeptide in the red cell membrane. The relationship of the encoding DNA exons and the amino acid residues differing between the Rh D and CcEe proteins are indicated.

Relationships Between Molecular Biology and Serological Reactivity

During 1994 and 1995, the *RHD* genes from partial and variant D individuals were cloned and sequenced. Two types were found – in some exons of the *RHD* gene appeared to have been substituted with the equivalent parts of the *RHCE* genes, producing hybrid *RHD/RHCE* genes [28]; in others point mutations were apparent in the *RHD* gene sequence [29]. These are shown diagrammatically in Figure 2. If the gene changes are superimposed on the model for Rh structure, one can predict which Rh D specific residues are changed in each variant, and which extracellular loops of the protein are affected. Examples of D^{Va} and D^{VI} are shown in Figures 3 and 4 . In 1996, [30] we examined all this data together with the reaction patterns of the monoclonal antibodies with the D variants see Table 4. Although the reaction patterns of some monoclonal antibodies could be explained on the basis of their interaction with D specific amino acids present in only one of the extracellular loops, many reaction patterns could only be explained by the antibody requiring D specific residues

Examples of Gene Structure of D variants

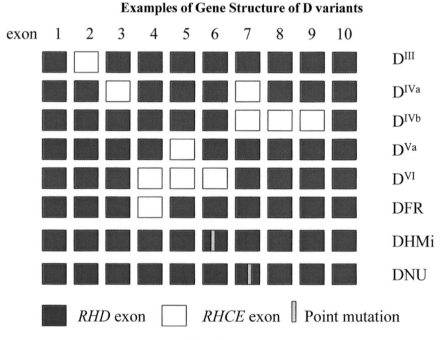

Fig. 2. Diagrammatic representation of the hybrid genes or point mutations responsible for partial D antigens.

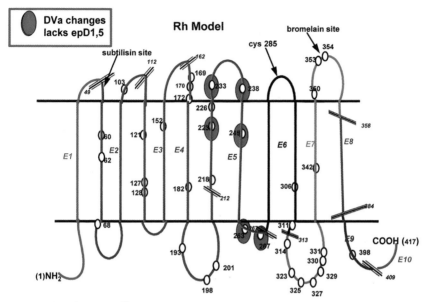

Fig. 3. Model of the Rh D^{Va} polypeptide in the red cell membrane. The relationship of the encoding DNA exons and the amino acid residues differing between the Rh D and CcEe proteins are indicated. The residues differing from a normal Rh D protein are highlighted.

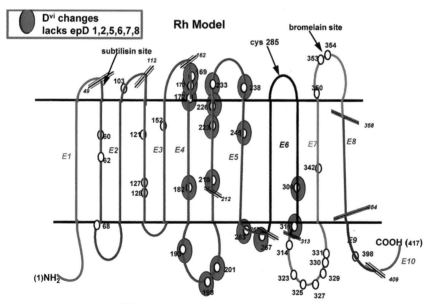

Fig. 4. Model of the Rh D^{VI} polypeptide in the red cell membrane. The relationship of the encoding DNA exons and the amino acid residues differing between the Rh D and CcEe proteins are indicated. The residues differing from a normal Rh D protein are highlighted.

Table 4. Exon changes and epitope loss in partial D phenotypes

Phenotype	Residues Changed	Exons Changed	Predicted Exofacial Loops Affected	Predicted exofacial residues affected	Epitopes lost
IIIb	60, 68, 103	2	2	103	27
IVa	62	2			1, 2, 3, 4, 5, 23, 26, 29, 30
	152	3			
	350	7	6	350	
IVb	350, 353, 354	7	6	350, 353, 354	1, 2, 3, 4, 5, 6, 23, 26, 29, 30
	398	9			
Va	223, 233, 238, 245, 263, 267	5	4	233, 238	1, 2, 8, 9, 10, 11, 26
VI	169, 170, 172, 182, 193, 198, 201,	4	3	169, 170, 172	1, 2, 3, 4, 7, 8, 9, 10, 11, 12, 13, 14, 15, 16, 17, 18, 19, 20, 21, 22, 26, 27, 28
	223, 233, 238, 245, 263, 267	5	4	233, 238	
	306, 311	6			
VII	110	2	2	110	22, 27, 28
DBT	218, 223, 226, 233, 238, 245, 263, 267	5	4	233, 238	1, 2, 3, 4, 5, 6, 7, 8, 9, 10, 11, 14, 15, 16, 19, 20, 21, 23, 25, 26, 27, 28, 29 30
	306, 311	6			
	314, 323, 325, 327, 329, 330, 331, 342, 350, 353, 354	7	6	350, 353, 354	

Table 4. *Continued.*

Phenotype	Residues Changed	Exons Changed	Predicted Exofacial Loops Affected	Predicted exofacial residues affected	Epitopes lost
DFR	169, 170, 172	4	3	169, 170, 171	2, 4, 9, 10, 11, 17, 18, 19, 20, 21, 22, 26, 27, 28
HAR	60, 62, 68, 103	2	2	103	1, 2, 3, 4, 5, 6, 8, 10, 11, 13, 15, 16, 18, 20, 21, 22, 23, 25, 26, 27, 28, 29, 30
	121, 127, 128, 152	3			
	169, 170, 172, 182, 193, 198, 201	4	3	169, 170, 172	
	306, 311	6			
	314, 323, 325, 327, 329, 330, 331	7	6	350, 353, 354	
	342, 350, 353, 354				
	398	9			

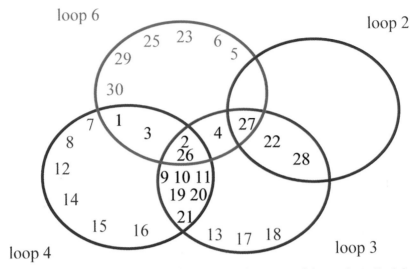

Fig. 5. Diagrammatic representation of the proposed position of the serologically defined Rh D epitopes relative to the extracellular loops of the protein.

in more than one of the extracellular loops. This hypothesis is shown diagrammatically in Figure 5. Such modelling cannot be prescriptive, as it is based on the study of the loss of D epitopes in knockout mutants. It cannot be assumed that the molecular changes associated with the epitope deficiencies are directly responsible for their expression. Changes in one region of the Rh D protein may affect other domains, and the introduction of bulky or charged side chains on external facing amino acids may significantly alter D antigenicity. In addition, few partial D phenotypes involve just one amino acid change; thus it is difficult to correlate the loss of a particular D epitope with a specific amino acid.

Site Directed Mutagenesis Studies

cDNA's encoding the Rh D and RH CcEe proteins have been expressed in the erythroleukaemia cell line K562, and the cells shown to react with Rh specific monoclonal antibodies by flow cytometry and immunofluorescent staining [31]. We have applied site directed mutagenesis to Rh cDNA's, then expressed these novel cDNA's in K562 cells and examined the cells for the expression of the different Rh D epitopes by staining with monoclonal antibodies specific for the different epitopes. In this way we have been able to examine the roles of different Rh D specific amino acid residues in the expression of the epitopes [32, 33].

Initially we examined the Rh D specific residues that are predicted to be exposed on extracellular loop 6 – residues Asp350, Ala353 and Gly354. Starting with an Rh cE cDNA, we introduced these three D specific residues by inverse PCR using mutagenic primers. Starting with Rh D cDNA, we introduced the equivalent RHCE coded residues (His350, Trp353 and Asn354). The constructs were introduced into a retroviral expression vector (pBabe) that confers puromycin resistance. After transduction of K562 cells, puromycin resistant clones were assessed for Rh D epitope expression, using monoclonal antibodies for indirect immunofluorescent staining and detection by flow cytometry. The results showed that the Rh D protein with CE residues in loop 6 showed identical monoclonal antibody binding to that observed with D^{IVb} cells, demonstrating that our SDM and expression approach could generate an Rh D antigen with identical binding properties to a naturally occurring Rh D variant antigen. In addition, the RH cE protein with D residues in loop 6 was able to bind 5 monoclonal anti-D with epD3 and epD9 specificities. This demonstrated that these particular monoclonal antibodies only require D specific residues in loop 6, whereas the other monoclonal antibodies must require critical residues in other loops [32].

A further six constructs were made, based on the Rh cE sequence, and incorporating D specific residues in loop 3, loop 4, loops 3 + 4, loops 3 + 6, loops 4 + 6 and loops 3 + 4 + 6. Table 5 shows the resulting patterns of reactivity with monoclonal antibodies.

On the basis of this data we have proposed a model for the arrangement of the Rh D protein in the red cell membrane (Figure 6) [33]. This model takes account of the possible physical size of an anti-D paratope (i.e. binding site) being no more than 20 Å in diameter. We thus assume that loops 3/4 and 4/6 must be in close proximity. Furthermore we suggest that loops 3 and 6 are non-adjacent, as no D epitopes were dependent on these two loops together. The model concludes that there are at least six conformationally different regions of the Rh D protein that are involved in D epitope expression.

Conclusions

Our D epitope cluster model is at present only a two-dimensional representation of D epitopes. Until highly resolved crystal structures of Rh D proteins with bound anti-D are obtained, the precise dimensions of D epitopes will remain speculative. However, it is clear that these dimensions will range from simple one loop structures, comprising linear stretches of amino acids (continuous epitopes) to highly conformation dependent discontinuous epitopes requiring interactions with residues in three or four different loops.

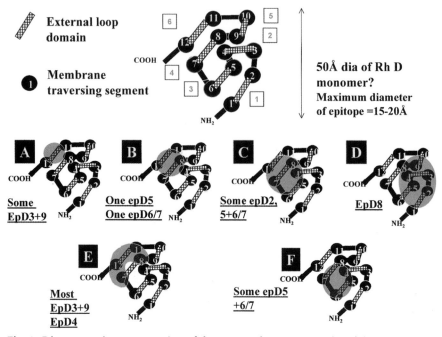

Fig. 6. Diagrammatic representation of the proposed 2-D topography of the extracellular loops of the Rh D polypeptide, and the location of the serologically defined Rh D epitopes.

Thus the high serological complexity of the Rh D antigen, demonstrated by the presence of the many naturally occurring variants and the differing fine specificities of monoclonal anti-D, can be explained by changes in nine critical extracellular residues of the protein, present on four extracellular loops. As with most antigen-antibody interactions, two to four residues of the paratope and epitope are required to interact to give rise to demonstrable binding, and the epitope residues can either be on one loop, or scattered across two, three or four loops that are close together in the tertiary conformation of the Rh D protein. Given this combinatorial picture it is not surprising that 24 epitopes have already been defined serologically – if three residues are critical for every binding then there are theoretically 84 different possible combinations! Constraint in the numbers is probably dependent on the span of the antibody paratope and the configuration of the loops in the membrane. Such is the nature of fine serological specificity, that changes in just one residue of the antigen or the antibody can determine whether binding occurs.

Table 5. Examples of flow cytometry immunoflorescent staining patterns with SDM cell lines

Epitope 1-9	Epitope 1-37	Antibody	cE	D	cE D loop 3	cE D loop 3+6	cE D loop 4	cE D loop 4+6	cE D loop 3+4	cE D loop 3+4+6	cE D loop 6
epD2	3	L871G7	4.2	**22.9**	4.2	3.4	3.7	6.7	4.1	**24.1**	4.2
epD3	5	LOR29	4.2	**20.1**	4.4	5.6	3.7	6.7	4.1	**23.3**	3.7
epD3	5	LHM76/55	4.3	**29.4**	4.3	5.9	4.0	**30.8**	4.2	**32.3**	3.4
epD3	5	LHM76/59	5.9	**25.3**	5.4	**27.7**	5.0	**51.7**	5.0	**27.0**	**14.9**
epD4	6	LOR176C7	3.7	**6.6**	3.8	3.1	3.2	**8.0**	4.1	**10.5**	3.6
epD5	8	D10	5.6	**35.7**	5.3	3.7	4.6	6.8	5.0	**21.7**	3.5
epD5	11	HAM.A	4.1	**17.1**	2.4	2.8	3.2	3.0	**20.2**	**25.0**	2.6
epD6/7	12	P3AF6	6.5	**30.9**	6.5	6.6	5.1	7.8	**26.2**	30.6	5.2
epD6/7	12	175-2	3.0	**13.4**	2.8	6.2	5.7	**24.4**	**15.8**	**17.5**	2.3
epD6/7	13	BRAD-3	4.1	**21.4**	2.6	6.7	2.9	3.3	7.5	**21.9**	3.0
epD6/7	15	D-90/7	5.1	**35.2**	5.5	3.8	4.5	5.2	4.7	**20.6**	3.4
epD6/7	17	P3 187	3.3	**18.8**	4.1	4.7	9.9	**30.6**	**22.6**	**21.2**	3.8
epD6/7	18	T3A2F6	6.4	**32.6**	3.5	**11.6**	6.4	2.4	**54.5**	**50.7**	**7.5**
epD6/7	19	MAD-2	5.1	**20.2**	3.1	3.6	3.4	3.9	**37.5**	**51.6**	3.1
epD6/7	21	HIRO-2	7.6	**20.2**	6.4	6.6	5.0	5.1	**16.5**	**18.9**	**7.4**
epD9	23	Birma D6	4.6	**30.4**	4.2	**32.7**	3.9	**52.4**	4.2	**29.0**	**13.1**
epD9	23	P3G6	4.2	**26.6**	3.9	5.0	3.5	**15.8**	4.0	**20.4**	2.9
epD9	30	8D8	4.9	**25.3**	5.8	9.3	5.4	**40.8**	4.9	**25.7**	**8.4**

Results shown are the mean fluorescent intensity. Positive results are in bold.

References

1. Levine P, Stetson RE (1939) An unusual case of intra-group agglutination. J Am Med Ass 113:126–127
2. Landsteiner K, Wiener AS (1940) An agglutinable factor in human blood recognised by immune sera for rhesus blood. Proc Soc Exp Biol NY 43:223
3. Landsteiner K, Wiener AS (1941) Studies on an agglutinogen (Rh) in human blood reacting with anti-rhesus sera and with human isoantibodies. J Exp Med 74:309–320
4. Wiener AS, Peters HR (1940) Hemolytic transfusion reactions following transfusion of blood of the homologous group, with three cases in which the same agglutinogen was responsible. Ann Int Med 13:2306–2322
5. Levine P, Burnham L, Katzin EM, Vogel P (1941) The role of iso-immunization in the pathogenesis of erythroblastosis fetalis. Am J Obst Gynecol 42:925–947
6. Fisk RT, Foord AG (1942) Observations on the Rh agglutinogen of human blood. Am J Clin Path 12:545
7. Levine P, Celano MJ, Wallace J, Sanger R (1963) A human "D-like" antibody. Nature 198:596–597
8. Wiener AS (1943) Genetic theory of the Rh blood types. Proc Soc Exp Biol Med 54:316–319
9. Levine P, Katzin EM, Burnham L (1941) Isoimmunization in pregnancy. Its possible bearing on the etiology of erythroblastosis foetalis. J Am Med Ass 116:825–827
10. Levine P, Vogel P, Katzin EM, Burnham L (1941) Pathogenesis of erythroblastosis fetalis: statistical evidence. Science 94:371–372
11. Mollinson PL, Engelfriet CP, Contreras M (1993) "Blood Transfusion in Clinical Medicine" 9th edition pp 111, 211 and 225. Blackwell Scientific Publications, Oxford,UK.
12. Argall CI, Ball JM, Trentleman E (1953) Presence of anti-D antibody in the serum of a D^u patient. J Lab Clin Med 41:895–898
13. Wiener AS, Unger U (1962) Further observations on blood factors Rh^A, Rh^B, Rh^C and Rh^D. Transfusion 2: 230–233
14. Tippett P, Sanger R (1962) Observations on subdivisions of the Rh antigen D. Vox Sang 7: 9–13
15. Lomas C, Grassman W, Ford D, Watt J, Gooch A, Jones J, Beolet M, Stern D, Wallace M, Tippett P (1994) FPTT is a low-incidence Rh antigen associated with a "new" partial D phenotype, DFR. Transfusion 34:612–616
16. Wallace M, Lomas-Francis C, Beckers E, Bruce M, Campbell G, Chatfield S, Nagao N, Okubo Y, Opalka A, Overbeeke M, Scott M, Voak D. (1997) DBT: a partial D phenotype associated with the low incidence antigen Rh32. Transfusion Medicine 7: 233–238
17. Lomas C, McColl K, Tippett P.(1993) Further complexities of the Rh antigen D disclosed by testing category D^{II} cells with monoclonal anti-D Transfusion Medicine 3:67–69
18. Jones J. (1993) Identification of two new variant D types using monoclonal anti-D reagents. Transfusion Medicine 3 (suppl 1):96
19. Scott ML (1996) Rh serology – Co-ordinator's report. Transfusion Clinique et Biologique 6: 333–338
20. Moore S, Woodrow CF, McLelland DB (1982) Isolation of membrane components associated with the human red cell antigens Rh (D), (c), (E) and Fy^a Nature 295:529–531

21. Saboori AM, Smith BL, Agre P (1988) Polymorphism in the Mr 32,000 Rh protein purified from Rh (D) positive and Rh (D) negative erythrocytes. Proc Natl Acad Sci USA 85:4042–4045

22. Blanchard D, Bloy C, Hermand P, Cartron J-P, Saboori AM, Smith BL, Agre P. (1988) Blood 72:1424–1427

23. Avent ND, Ridgwell K, Tanner MJA, Anstee DJ (1990) cDNA cloning of a 30 kDa erythrocyte membrane protein associated with Rh (rhesus) blood group antigen expression. Biochem J 271:821–825

24. Cherif-Zahar B, Bloy C, Le Van Kim C, Blanchard D, Bailly P, Hermand P, Salmon C, Cartron J-P, Colin Y (1990) Molecular cloning and protein structure of a human blood group Rh polypeptide. Proc Natl Acad Sci USA 87:6243–6247

25. Le van Kim C, Mouro I, Cherif-Zahar B, Raynal V, Cherrier V, Cartron J-P, Colin Y. (1992) Molecular cloning and primary structure of the human blood group Rh D polypeptide. Proc Natl Acad Sci USA 89:10925–10929

26. Colin Y, Cherif-Zahar B, Le van Kim C, Raynal V, van Huffel V, Cartron J-P (1991) Genetic basis of the Rh D positive and Rh D negative blood group polymorphism as determined by Southern analysis. Blood 78:2747–2752

27. Cherif-Zahar B, Le van Kim C, Rouillac C, Raynal V, Cartron J-P, Colin Y (1994) Organisation of the gene RHCE encoding the Rh CcEe antigens and characterisation of the promoter region. Genomics 19:68–74

28. Mouro I, Le van Kim C, Rouillac C, van Rhenen D, Le Pennec PY, Cartron J-P, Colin Y. (1994) Rearrangements of the blood group Rh D gene associated with the D–VI category. Blood 83:1129–1134

29. Liu W, Jones JW, Scott ML, Voak D, Avent ND (1996) Molecular analysis of two D variants – DHMi and DHMii. Transfusion Med 6 suppl 2 :21. (Abstract)

30. Scott ML, Voak D, Jones JW, Avent ND, Liu W, Hughes-Jones NC, Sonneborn H (1996) A structural model for 30 Rh D epitopes based on serological and DNA sequence data from partial D phenotypes. Transfusion Clinique et Biologique 6:391–396

31. Smythe JS, Avent ND, Judson PA, Parsons SF, Martin PG, Anstee DJ (1996). Expression of RHD and RHCE gene products using retroviral transduction of K562 cells establishes the molecular basis of Rh blood group antigens. Blood 87: 2968–2973

32. Liu W, Smythe JS, Scott ML, Voak D, Avent N. (1999) Site directed mutagenesis of the human Rh D antigen: definition of D epitopes on the sixth external domain of the D protein expressed on K562 cells. Transfusion 39:17–25

33. Liu W, Avent ND, Jones JW, Scott ML, Voak D. (1999) Molecular configuration of RH D epitopes as defined by site-directed mutagenesis and expression of mutant RH constructs in K562 erythroleukaemia cells. Blood 94: 3986–3996

CHAPTER 6

Infections and the Immune Response to Cardiac Antigens

J. M. Penninger[1] and K. Bachmaier[1]

Abstract

Cardiovascular disease is predicted to be the commonest cause of death worldwide by the year 2020, and heart disease remains the most prevalent cause of morbidity and mortality in rich countries. In recent years, infections with various pathogens have emerged as risk factors for cardiovascular disease. While a causal dependence has not yet been established, experimental animal models were useful to gain insights into potential mechanisms linking infectious agents to the pathogenesis of heart disease: Cytopathic effects of cardiotropic viruses can trigger autoimmune responses to heart-specific epitopes. Autoaggressive lymphocytes can be activated by mimicking peptides present in diverse and common human-pathogenic bacteria. Autoinflammatory processes induce perivascular inflammation, fibrotic changes, and blood vessel occlusion in the heart. Inflammatory cardiomyopathy leads to dilated cardiomyopathy, the principal condition necessitating heart transplantation. Considering autoinflammatory mechanisms will have important implications on diagnostic and therapeutic strategies for cardiovascular diseases.

Introduction

Clinical as well as experimental studies imply that chronic stages of various heart diseases are, at least in part, mediated by autoimmune responses to cardiac antigens (Rose, 1996). Inflammatory heart disease can be caused by a wide variety of pathogens such as viruses, bacteria and protozoa (Rose, 1996; Woodruff, 1980). RNA of the Picornavirus Coxsackie B3 (CVB3), one of the viruses responsible for the common cold, can be detected in the heart muscle

[1] Amgen Institute, Ontario Cancer Institute, Department of Medical Biophysics, University of Toronto, 620 University Avenue, Suite 706, Toronto, Ontario M5G 2C1, Canada

in up to 50 % of patients with dilated cardiomyopathy (DCM) defined by enlargement of cardiac chambers, thinning of ventricular walls, and reduced myofibrillar contractility (Dec et al., 1985; Fenoglio et al., 1983; James, 1983; Keating and Sanguinetti, 1996). Since almost all people have been infected with CVB3 and harbor anti-CVB3 antibodies it appears that CVB3 might induce myocarditis very frequently in human populations without ever being diagnosed (Martino, 1994). Who would perform endomyocardial biopsies in patients with a common cold? Infections with another common human pathogen, *Chlamydia pneumoniae* are epidemiologically linked to human heart disease and *C. psittaci* and *C. trachomatis* infections have been shown to lead directly to endocarditis or myocarditis. *Chlamydia* infections also cause pneumonia, conjunctivitis in children, and are a primary cause of sexually transmitted diseases and female infertility (Danesh et al., 1997; Grayston et al., 1981; Munoz and West, 1997; Odeh et al., 1991; Ossewaarde et al., 1998; Saikku et al., 1988; Stokes, 1997). A peptide from the murine heart muscle-specific α myosin heavy chain that has sequence homology to the 60-kilodalton cysteine-rich outer membrane proteins of Chlamydia pneumoniae, C. psittaci, and C. trachomatis induces autoimmune inflammatory heart disease in mice. Injection of the homologous Chlamydia peptides into mice also induced perivascular inflammation, fibrotic changes, and blood vessel occlusion in the heart, as well as triggering T and B cell reactivity to the homologous endogenous heart muscle-specific peptide (Bachmaier et al., 1999). Infection with C. trachomatis leads to the production of autoantibodies to heart muscle-specific epitopes and perivascular inflammation (Bachmaier et al., 1999; Fan et al., 1999). Thus, we concluded that Chlamydia-mediated heart disease was induced by antigenic mimicry of a heart muscle-specific protein. However, studies designed to reveal a correlation between future risk of heart disease and Chlamydia infection have been inconclusive (Anderson et al., 1999; Ridker et al., 1999). While these results mitigated against the "infection hypothesis", they may not have been surprising since bacteria other than Chlamydia, i.e., B*orrelia burgdorferi, Treponema pallidum, Mycoplasma pneumoniae,* and *Mycoplasma genitalium* also supply mimicking epitopes (Bachmaier et al., 2000). Infections with common human pathogens may be causative in heart disease. Thus, identifying the subsets of patients at risk of progression from acute infections to chronic cardiomyopathy, will be crucial. The challenge will be to determine both genetic and environmental factors that govern the progression to chronic heart disease and the development of DCM. Inflammatory heart disease in humans can be experimentally reproduced in mice to analyze the interplay between host and pathogens.

The Murine Model of Experimental Autoimmune Myocarditis

The development of a murine model of autoimmune myocarditis was based on genetic differences among inbred mouse strains in the immune response to Coxsackie virus B3 (CVB3)-induced myocarditis (Neu et al., 1987). In certain mouse strains CVB3 mediated myocarditis evolves in an early phase characterized by myocyte damage due to CVB3 cytotoxicity during acute viral infection and a late phase that is associated with the production of heart muscle specific auto-antibodies and inflammatory infiltration of T cells, B cells and macrophages into the myocardium (Neu et al., 1987; Rose et al., 1988). The Src-family kinase p56^{lck} is required for efficient CVB3 replication in T cell lines and for viral replication and persistence in mice, identifying p56^{lck} as a crucial host factor that controls the replication and pathogenicity of CVB3 (Liu et al., 2000). Moreover, mice deficient for the tyrosine phosphatase CD45 are completely protected from lethal CVB3 infections and do not show any histological lesions of acute or chronic inflammation in the heart, pancreas, liver or brain. Thus, the loss of CD45 renders mice resistant to lethal infections with CVB3 (Irie-Sasaki et al., 2001). The later phase of CVB3 induced heart disease can be mimicked by immunization of mice with purified murine cardiac myosin in the absence of virus infection and experimental cardiac myosin-induced myocarditis has immunological and histopathological features that resemble postviral heart disease in mice and dilated cardiomyopathy in humans (Neu et al., 1987; Rose et al., 1988).

A Genetic Approach to Autoimmune Myocarditis

Mouse Experimental Autoimmune Myocarditis Is a T cell-Mediated Disease

In experimental autoimmune myocarditis, the inflammatory infiltrate consists of CD4$^+$ T cells, (~10 %), CD8$^+$ T cells (~5–7 %), few B cells (~1–2 %) with local deposition of heart muscle protein-specific auto-Ab, and CD11b$^+$ macrophages (70–80 % of infiltrating cells) (Pummerer et al., 1991). Inflammation of the heart muscle can be transferred into non-immunized recipient mice by purified T cells from mice with active myocarditis (Bachmaier et al., 1997; Pummerer et al., 1996). Autoimmune heart disease does not occur in mice lacking the Src-family tyrosine kinase p56^{lck} or the tyrosine phosphatase CD45 which regulates the enzymatic activity of p56^{lck} (Table 1) (Bachmaier et al., 1996). Mice lacking CD8 after gene targeting develop a significantly more severe disease as compared to heterozygous littermates implying that CD8$^+$ lymphocytes do not only act as cytotoxic effector cells in autoimmunity but may also regulate disease severity. Remarkably, CD4-deficient mice also develop mild

Table 1. Prevalence and severity of experimental autoimmune myocarditis in transgenic mice in comparison to wild-type controls

Genotype	Prevalence	Disease severity
p56$^{lck-/-}$	no disease	–
p56$^{lck+/-}$	high	severe
CD45$^{-/-}$	no disease	–
CD45$^{+/-}$	high	severe
CD4$^{+/-}$8$^{+/-}$	high	severe
CD4$^{-/-}$	intermediate	mild
CD8$^{-/-}$	high	severe
CD28$^{+/-}$	high	severe
CD28$^{-/-}$	low	mild
TNF-Rp55$^{-/-}$	no disease	–
TNF-Rp55$^{+/-}$	high	severe
IRF-1$^{-/-}$	high	severe
IRF-1$^{+/-}$	high	severe
IRF-2$^{-/-}$	high	severe
IRF-2$^{+/-}$	high	severe
hCD4TG	low	mild
hCD4/DQ6TG	high	severe

autoimmune myocarditis characterized by a high proportion of TCR$_{\alpha\beta}^+$CD4$^-$CD8$^-$ infiltrating cells (Table 1) (Penninger et al., 1993). Animals that lack the T cell costimulatory molecule CD28 develop disease at significantly lower severity and prevalence as compared to control littermates and showed a defect in (Th2 mediated) IgG1 auto-Ab production (Table 1) (Bachmaier et al., 1996).

The Role of Antigen Presenting Cells

"Professional" antigen presenting cells (APC) located within the myocardium are the primary target of autoreactive T cells during the initial phases of autoimmune heart disease. Heart APCs process and present antigens derived from cardiac myosin (Smith and Allen, 1992). Expression of MHC class II molecules and other adhesion molecules such as ICAM-1 and CD31 both of which are predominantly expressed on endothelial cells precedes cellular infiltration of T lymphocytes into the heart. In vivo injection of mAbs against MHC class II molecules or injection of nonimmunogenic, competitor peptides that bind to MHC class II molecules can prevent autoimmune heart disease (Pummerer et al., 1991). In addition, the induction of autoimmune myocarditis is strain dependent and the MHC class II haplotype (such as H-2$^{k/k}$ in disease susceptible A/J mice or H-2$^{d/d}$ in susceptible Balb/c mice) is the single most important genetic factor to confer disease susceptibility (Neu et al., 1987; Penninger et al., 1996). Heart interstitial APCs from TNF-Rp55 deficient mice fail to upregulate MHC class II molecules after immunization with cardiac myosin. Upregulation of MHC class II molecules on heart interstitial cells has important functional consequences for the pathogenesis of autoimmunity since these mice are completely protected from autoimmune myocarditis (Table 1) (Bachmaier et al., 1997).

One of the consequences of inflammation in autoimmune heart disease is injury of cardiomyocytes and subsequent progression to heart failure and DCM. iNOS expression has been found in the myocardium of DCM patients and patients with ischemic heart disease or valvular heart disease (Habib et al., 1996; Haywood et al., 1996). iNOS expression, elicited in inflammatory macrophages and in heart muscle cells in autoimmune heart disease in mice, is accompanied by formation of the NO reaction product nitrotyrosine in inflammatory macrophages as well as in virtually all heart muscle cells. Remarkably, already weak focal inflammation induces nitrosylation of tyrosine residues on heart muscle proteins of the whole heart. IRF-1 is the crucial transcription factor for iNOS expression in macrophages and cardiomyocytes during autoimmune inflammation since mice defective for IRF-1 fail to express iNOS protein and do not show any nitrotyrosine formation in the heart muscle or infiltrating macrophages (Bachmaier et al., 1997). Recently, it has been shown that IFN-γ receptor-deficient mice on a BALB/c background develop severe autoimmune myocarditis, upon experimental immunization, with high mortality. IFN-γ possibly protects mice from lethal autoimmune myocarditis by inducing the expression of iNOS followed by the downregulation of T-cell responses (Eriksson et al., 2001).

"Humanized" Mice Susceptible
to Autoimmune Inflammatory Heart Disease

Chronic heart diseases in humans have been linked to certain HLA alleles, such as HLA-DQ6. Using mice double CD4- and CD8-deficient and transgenic for human CD4 (hCD4) and human HLA-DQ6 to specifically reconstitute the human CD4/DQ6 arm of the immune system in mice, we provided experimental evidence showing that human MHC class II molecules are involved in the pathogenesis of myocarditis and DCM. Transgenic hCD4 and HLA-DQ6 expression rendered genetically resistant C57BL/6 mice susceptible to the induction of autoimmune myocarditis induced by immunization with cardiac myosin (Table 1) (Bachmaier et al., 1999). The autoimmune inflammatory heart disease induced by the human heart muscle specific peptide in hCD4 and HLA-DQ6 double transgenic mice shares functional and phenotypic features with the disease occurring in disease-susceptible non transgenic mice (Penninger et al., 1996).

Antigenic Mimicry

The in vivo mapping of endogenous immunodominant and heart-pathogenic epitopes preceded the detection of mimicking epitopes present in diverse bacteria. Confirmation of the importance of a pathogenic peptide motif present in the heart specific α myosin heavy chain in vivo provided the tools to find matching bacterial epitopes.

Heart Specific α-Myosin Heavy Chain-Derived Peptides With Major Pathogenicity

T cells recognize peptides presented by MHC class I or MHC class II molecules (June et al., 1994). Immunodominant peptides derived from the cardiac α-myosin heavy chain (αmhc) isoform have been identified that can induce autoimmune myocarditis in BALB/c (Pummerer et al., 1996) and A/J mice (Donermeyer et al., 1995). Alpha-myosin is the immunodominant isoform and induces myocarditis at high prevalence and severity whereas the β-myosin isoform induces little disease. Thus, the immunodominant epitopes had to reside within regions of different amino acid sequences between α- and β-myosin. Using this approach three pathogenic epitopes of α-myosin were mapped (Pummerer et al., 1996). One peptide is located in the head portion of the molecule (αmhc (614–643)) and induces severe myocarditis whereas two others in the rod portion of α-myosin possess only minor pathogenicity. In A/J mice the pathogenic epitope is located at a different region on the α-myosin molecule (amino acids 334–352) as compared to the immunodominant epitopes in BALB/c mice. Importantly, the same group also showed that this peptide binds strongly to I-A^k molecules and forms a stable complex with MHC class II molecules (Donermeyer et al., 1995). It should also be noted that two immunodominant cardiac myosin peptides (CM1: TRGKLSYTQQMEDLKRQ;

and CM2: KLELQSALEEAEASLEH) have been identified which can induce experimental myocarditis in rats (Wegmann et al., 1994).

Chlamydia Infections Lead to the Activation of Autoaggressive Lymphocytes Reactive to Heart-Specific Antigens

Infections with the common human pathogen Chlamydia pneumoniae are epidemiologically linked to human heart disease. We hypothesized that the mechanism by which Chlamydia causes cardiovascular disease might involve antigenic mimicry. The first 16 amino acids of the αmhc (614–643) peptide [αmhc (614–629)] constitute a dominant autoaggressive epitope, designated M7Aα (Table 2) (Bachmaier et al., 1999). In contrast, the homologous region of the β myosin heavy chain isoform, designated M7Aβ, does not induce disease (Table 2, Fig. 1A). Single amino acid substitutions into M7Aα further revealed the importance of the xxxMAxxxSTxxx motif for the pathogenicity of M7Aα in vivo. Peptide sequences from the 60-kD cysteine-rich outer membrane protein (CRP) from different serovars of C. trachomatis match the M7Aα motif, and are designated ChTR1 (serovar E), ChTR2 (serovar C), ChTR3 (serovars L1, L2 and L3). The homologous peptides from the 60-kD CRPs of C. pneumoniae, designated ChPN, and C. psittaci, designated ChPS, shared sequence identities with the M7Aα motif, albeit to a lesser extent (Table 2). All of these Chlamydia-derived peptides induce inflammatory heart disease at a similar frequency, albeit at significantly lower severity, as compared to M7Aα immunized mice (Table 2). Like the inflammation that follows immunization with the endogenous autoantigen M7Aα, the disease induced by the Chlamydia

Table 5.2. Prevalence and severity of autoimmune myocarditis induced by Chlamydia derived peptides that mimic a heart specific α-myosin heavy chain derived peptide

Peptide	Amino acid sequence	Prevalence	Severity
M7Aα	SLKLMATLFSTYASAD	high	high
CHTR1	VLETSMAEFTSTNVIS	high	mild
CHTR2	VLETSMAESLSTNVIS	high	mild
CHTR3	VLETSMAEFISTNVIS	high	mild
CHPN	GIEAAVAESLITKIVA	high	mild
CHPS	KIEAAAAESLATRFIA	high	mild
M7Aβ	SLKLLSNLFANYASAD	no disease	–

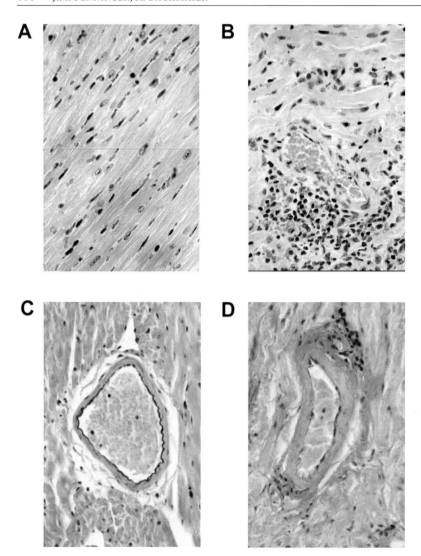

Fig. 1. A, B Heart histology in BALB/c mice that were immunized with (**A**) the control endogenous mouse peptide designated M7Aβ from the β myosin heavy chain; (**B**); the 60-kD Cystein rich outer membrane protein (CRP)-derived peptide from C. trachomatis (ChTR1) sharing the pathogenic peptide motif with the endogenous mouse peptide designated M7Aα from the α myosin heavy chain. Note the perivascular mononuclear inflammatory infiltrate. Hearts were analyzed 21 days after the initial immunization. H.&E. staining. Magnifications ×320   **C, D**   Blood vessels in mice immunized with M7Aβ or C. trachomatis 60-kD CRP-derived peptid. (**C**) Normal morphology of the cardiac artery in mice immunized with non-pathogenic M7Aβ. (**D**) Thickening of the arterial wall and perivascular fibrotic changes in mice immunized with ChTR1. Note the perivascular mononuclear inflammatory cells. Elastica staining for collagen (red) to detect fibrotic changes. Magnifications ×320.

Table 3. Parainfluenza virus 1 or Human immunodeficiency virus 2 derived peptides that mimic heart specific a-myosin heavy chain derived peptides do not induce autoimmune myocarditis

Peptide	Amino acid sequence	Prevalence	Severity
αmhc(314-332)	DSAFDVLSFTAEEKAGVYK	high	high
Parainfluenza virus 1 [HT83b] (291-309)	DLVFDILDLKGKTKSPRYK	no disease	–
αmhc (735-747)	GQFIDSGKGAEKL	low	intermediate
HIV2 [gp160]	INFIGPGKGSDPE	no disease	–

derived peptides is characterized by perivascular and pericardial infiltration of mononuclear cells and fibrotic changes (Fig. 1B). Mice immunized with Chlamydia peptides develop perivascular fibrosis (Fig. 1C, D), fibrinous occlusions of cardiac blood vessels and thickening of the arterial walls. The inflammatory infiltrate in ChTR1 peptide-induced heart disease is similar to cardiac myosin and cardiac myosin-derived peptide induced myocarditis, consisting of about 11 % $CD4^+$ and 12 % $CD8^+$ T cells, 16 % $B220^+$ B cells, and 61 % $CD11b^+$ macrophages. In contrast to the peptides matching the M7Aα motif, injection of mice with HIV2 or Parainfluenza virus 1 derived peptides that share homology with other immunogenic regions of the mouse αmhc molecule does not cause inflammatory heart disease (Table 3) (Bachmaier et al., 1999).

Splenic T cells from mice immunized with the endogenous peptide M7Aα proliferate when incubated with splenocytes pulsed with the M7Aα peptide. Splenic T cells from these mice also show a strong proliferative response to the C. trachomatis derived peptide ChTR1. Splenic T cells from mice immunized with ChTR1 proliferated to ChTR1 and to the endogenous M7Aα peptide. Thus, ChTR1 peptide immunizations can cross-prime for T cell reactivity against the endogenous M7Aα (Bachmaier et al., 1999). Murine autoimmune myocarditis is accompanied by the T cell-dependent production of autoantibodies to cardiac epitopes (Neu et al., 1987). Immunization with endogenous M7Aα peptide leads to the production of serum antibodies to the M7Aα peptide and to the ChTR1 peptide (Bachmaier et al., 1999). Likewise, immunization with the C. trachomatis-derived peptide ChTR1 induces the production of serum antibodies to ChTR1 and to the endogenous M7Aα peptide. Mice immunized with either M7Aα and ChTR1 also have antibodies to the kkα peptide, an unrelated heart specific peptide, suggesting that M7Aα and ChTR1 induced heart disease leads to epitope spreading at the B cell level.

Inflammation of both the respiratory tract or the reproductive organs caused by local C. trachomatis inocculation, leads to the production of IgG antibodies to heart-specific epitopes in BALB/c mice (Bachmaier et al., 1999). Because in the mouse model of autoimmune myocarditis, the production of IgG antibodies to heart-specific epitopes is dependent on the activation of autoaggressive T and B cells, these data showed that infection by C. trachomatis can activate autoaggressive lymphocytes in BALB/c mice. Moreover, pulmonary infection with C. trachomatis can induce myocardial and perivascular inflammation and fibrosis in C57BL/6 mice (Fan et al., 1999). Thus, antigenic mimicry of autoaggressive myosin epitopes by peptides present not only in C. pneumoniae but also in C. trachomatis and C. psittaci is linked to inflammatory heart disease.

Pathogenic Motifs Mimicking Heart Epitopes Are Prevalent in Diverse Bacteria

Studies designed to reveal a correlation between future risk of heart disease and Chlamydia infection have been inconclusive (Anderson et al., 1999; Ridker et al., 1999). While these results mitigate against the "infection hypothesis", they are not surprising if organisms other than Chlamydia also supply mimicking epitopes. Searching public databases revealed that the pathogenic mouse M7Aα peptide MAxxxST motif (see Table 1) is present in various human pathogens: Borrelia burgdorferi, the spirochete causing Lyme disease; Treponema pallidum, the causative agent of syphilis; Mycoplasma pneumoniae, an etiologic agent of non-viral primary atypical pneumonia; Mycoplasma genitalium, associated with urogenital infection; and Helicobacter pylori, associated with duodenal and gastric ulcers; as well as the protozoon Trypanosoma cruzi, the cause of Chagas disease. Remarkably, 5 out of the 9 microbial peptides examined induce inflammatory heart disease, albeit less severe than the endogenous heart-specific pathogenic peptide M7Aα (Table 4). Peptides derived from Borrellia burgdorferi, Treponema pallidum, Mycoplasma pneumoniae, and Mycoplasma genitalium induce inflammatory heart disease whereas peptides from Helicobacter pylori, and Trypanosoma cruzi fail to induce disease (Table 4).

Inflammatory heart disease is accompanied by T cell-dependent production of autoantibodies to cardiac epitopes and immunization of mice with the endogenous M7Aα peptide leads to the production of anti-M7Aα serum antibodies (Bachmaier et al., 1999). Induction of inflammatory heart disease by the microbial peptides examined in this study was also characterized by the production of serum autoantibodies reactive to M7Aα (Table 4). Immunization with peptides derived from diverse bacteria leads to the breaking of immuno-

Table 4. Sequence alignment of microbial peptides with the pathogenic mouse M7Aα and the non-pathogenic M7Aβ peptides. Prevalence, severity of inflammatory heart disease, and autoantibody titers in mice immunized with indicated peptides.

Peptide (Accession number)	Amino acid sequence diseased/immunized mice	Prevalence mean±SEM	Severity mean±SEM	Autoantibody titers
M7Aα (M76598)	SLKLMATLFSTYASA	5/5	2.6±0.3	640±55
Treponema pallidum (H71326)	RSEAMALVLSTLENR	4/5	1.3±0.1	280±27
Borrelia burgdorferi (Q44775)	LFLIMATFLSPSISG	4/5	1.5±0.1	400±61
Mycoplasma pneumonia (S73638)	SGQYIASHFSTHNEV	3/5	1.0±0.0	466±76
Mycoplasma pneumoniae (S62837)	TPPNMATLVSTAMSL	2/5	1.0±0.0	300±35
Mycoplasma genitalium (B64239)	TGQYMASFFSTNSEP	2/5	1.0±0.0	200±35
Helicobacter pylori (B40586)	TYNVMATGTSPVMSG	0/5	–	–
Helicobacter pylori (C64534)	DSSGMAIADSLRSQS	0/5	–	–
Helicobacter pylori (G64648)	IHDKMARNLSSQVSS	0/5	–	–
Trypanosoma cruzi (S27852)	NTFHMAGGGSTLINL	0/5	–	–
M7Aβ (P02564)	SLKLLSNLFANYASA	0/5	–	–

Six-week-old BALB/c mice were immunized with the indicated peptides [50 μg per mouse] in Freund's complete adjuvant (FCA), boosted 7 days later in the same manner, and analyzed 21 days after the initial immunization for the presence and severity of myocarditis. Histological grading of severity was as follows: 0, no lymphocytic infiltration into the heart muscle; 1, up to 5 % of the histological cross-section was infiltrated; 2, 6 to 10 %; 3, 11 to 20 %; 4>20 %. M7Aα, the murine α myosin heavy chain molecule (positive control); M7Aβ, rat β myosin heavy chain molecule (negative control). Letters in red indicate positions of sequence identity to M7Aα. For autoantibody titer determinations, sera were collected at the time of sacrifice and IgG reactive to M7Aα was measured by ELISA. The inverse of the highest serum dilution giving 0.1 absorption units above control values was taken as the titer. Mean value ± SEM is given for mice with myocarditis. Mice without myocarditis had autoantibody titres <50.

tolerance towards a defined heart-specific epitope, the activation of autoaggressive T and B lymphocytes, the production of autoantibodies and histopathological changes within the heart muscle and heart blood vessels. Thus, pathogenic motifs mimicking heart epitopes are prevalent in diverse bacteria. Interestingly, Borrelia burgdorferi, Treponema pallidum and Chlamydia trachomatis, all of which can provide epitopes mimicking heart-specific proteins, were discovered in specimen collected from the subgingival flora of an apparently healthy 39-year old male (Kroes et al., 1999). The immune system's response to a mimicking epitope depends on the genetic background of the host explaining why not all of us develop cardiovascular disease after suffering microbial infections. Murine and human M7Aα epitopes are evolutionarily conserved, and human MHC class II molecules and human heart muscle-specific autoantigens such as M7Aα can cause inflammatory heart disease (Bachmaler et al., 1999). Not only Chlamydia can provide mimicking epitopes but these epitopes are present in diverse bacteria. Molecular mimicry between bacterial and viral proteins and endogenous molecules has been implicated in various autoimmune diseases, including insulin-dependent diabetes, multiple sclerosis, and autoimmune herpes stromal keratitis. After initiation of the disease, epitope spreading leads to maintenance and progression of inflammation. Other mechanisms that could also contribute to the pathogenesis of cardiovascular diseases after microbial infection include the production of inflammatory cytokines, bystander activation of lymphocytes, or both (Horwitz et al., 1998; Janeway CA, 1998; Oldstone, 1987; Zabriskie and Friedman, 1983). Our results on antigenic mimicry between bacterial and endogenous heart peptides also imply that the microbes do not have to be present within the heart, and inflammation, caused by diverse bacteria, outside the heart might be sufficient to trigger and/or could contribute to heart disease.

The challenge for the development of successful prevention and treatment strategies will be to diagnose those at risk to develop severe heart disease among the many with microbial infections.

References

Anderson JL, Muhlestein JB, Carlquist J, Allen A, Trehan S, Nielson C, Hall S, Brady J, Egger M, Horne B, Lim T (1999). Randomized secondary prevention trial of azithromycin in patients with coronary artery disease and serological evidence for Chlamydia pneumoniae infection: The Azithromycin in Coronary Artery Disease: Elimination of Myocardial Infection with Chlamydia (ACADEMIC) study [see comments]. Circulation 99,1540–1547

Bachmaier K, Le J, Penninger JM (2000) "Catching heart disease": antigenic mimicry and bacterial infections [letter]. Nat Med 6, 841–842

Bachmaier K, Neu N, de la Maza LM, Pal S, Hessel A, Penninger JM (1999) Chlamydia infections and heart disease linked through antigenic mimicry [see comments]. Science 283, 1335–1339

Bachmaier K, Neu N, Pummerer C, Duncan GS, Mak TW, Matsuyama T, Penninger JM (1997) iNOS expression and nitrotyrosine formation in the myocardium in response to inflammation is controlled by the interferon regulatory transcription factor 1. Circulation. 96, 585–591

Bachmaier K, Neu N, Yeung RSM, Mak TW, Liu P, Penninger JM (1999) Generation of humanized mice susceptible to peptide-induced inflammatory heart disease. Circulation 99, 1885–1891

Bachmaier K, Pummerer C, Kozieradzki I, Pfeffer K, Mak TW, Neu N, Penninger JM (1997) Low-molecular-weight tumor necrosis factor receptor p55 controls induction of autoimmune heart disease. Circulation 95, 655–661

Bachmaier K, Pummerer C, Shahinian A, Ionescu J, Neu N, Mak TW, Penninger JM (1996) Induction of autoimmunity in the absence of CD28 costimulation. J Immunol 157, 1752–1757

Danesh J, Collins R, Peto R (1997) Chronic infections and coronary heart disease: is there a link? Lancet 350, 430–436

Dec GW Jr, Palacios IF, Fallon JT, Aretz HT, Mills J, Lee DC, Johnson RA (1985) Active myocarditis in the spectrum of acute dilated cardiomyopathies. Clinical features, histologic correlates, and clinical outcome. New Engl Med. 312, 885–890

Donermeyer DL, Beisel KW, Allen PM, Smith SC (1995) Myocarditis-inducing epitope of myosin binds constitutively and stably to I-A(k) on antigen-presenting cells in the heart. Exp Med. 182, 1291–1300

Eriksson U, Kurrer MO, Bingisser R, Eugster HP, Saremaslani P, Follath F, Marsch S, Widmer U (2001) Lethal autoimmune myocarditis in interferon-gamma receptor-deficient mice: enhanced disease severity by impaired inducible nitric oxide synthase induction. Circulation (Online) 103, 18–21

Fan Y, Wang S, Yang X (1999) Chlamydia trachomatis (mouse pneumonitis strain) induces cardiovascular pathology following respiratory tract infection. Infect Immun 67, 6145–6151

Fenoglio JJ Jr, Ursell PC, Kellogg CF, Drusin RE, Weiss MB (1983) Diagnosis and classification of myocarditis by endomyocardial biopsy. N Engl J Med 308, 12–18

Grayston JT, Mordhorst CH, Wang SP (1981) Childhood myocarditis associated with Chlamydia trachomatis infection. JAMA 246, 2823–2827

Habib FM, Springall DR, Davies GJ, Oakley CM, Yacoub MH, Polak JM (1996) Tumour necrosis factor and inducible nitric oxide synthase in dilated cardiomyopathy [see comments]. Lancet 347, 1151–1155

Haywood GA, Tsao PS, von der Leyen HE, Mann MJ, Keeling PJ, Trindade PT, Lewis NP, Byrne CD, Rickenbacher PR, Bishopric NH, Cooke JP, McKenna WJ, Fowler MB (1996). Expression of inducible nitric oxide synthase in human heart failure [see comments]. Circulation 93, 1087–1094

Horwitz MS, Bradley LM, Harbertson J, Krahl T, Lee J, Sarvetnick N (1998) Diabetes induced by Coxsackie virus: Initiation by bystander damage and not molecular mimicry. Nature Med 4, 781–785

Irie-Sasaki J, Sasaki T, Matsumoto W, Opavsky A, Cheng M, Welstead G, Griffiths E, Krawczyk C, Richardson CD, Aitken K, Iscove N, Koretzky G, Johnson P, Liu P, Rothstein DM, Penninger JM (2001). CD45 is a JAK phosphatase and negatively regulates cytokine receptor signalling. Nature. 409, 349–354

James TN (1983) Myocarditis and cardiomyopathy [editorial]. N Engl J Med 308, 39–41

Janeway CA (1998) A tale of two T cells. Immunity 8, 391–394

June CH, Bluestone JA, Nadler LM, Thompson CB (1994) The B7 and CD28 receptor families. Immunol Today 15, 321–331

Keating MT, Sanguinetti MC (1996) Molecular genetic insights into cardiovascular disease. Science 272, 681–685

Kroes I, Lepp PW, Relman DA (1999) Bacterial diversity within the human subgingival crevice. Proc Natl Acad Sci USA 96, 14547–14552

Liu P, Aitken K, Kong YY, Martino T, Dawood F, Wen WH, Opavsky MA, Kozieradzki I, Bachmaier K, Straus D, Mak TW, Penninger JM (2000) Essential role for the tyrosine kinase p56lck in Coxsackievirus B3-mediated heart disease. Nature Med 6(4):429–34

Martino TA, Liu P, Sole MJ (1994) Viral infection and the pathogenesis of dilated cardiomyopathy. Circ. Res. 74, 182–188

Munoz B, West S (1997) Trachoma: the forgotten cause of blindness. Epidemiol Rev 19, 205–217

Neu N, Craig SW, Rose NR et al. (1987) Coxsackievirus induced myocarditis in mice: Cardiac myosin autoantibodies do not cross-react with the virus. Clinical and Experimental Immunology. 69, 566–574

Neu N, Rose NR, Beisel KW, Herskowitz A, Gurro G-G, Craig SW (1987) Cardiac myosin induces myocarditis in genetically predisposed mice. Journal of Immunology. 139, 3630–3636

Odeh M, Oliven A, Rauchfleisch S, Bassan H (1991) Dilated cardiomyopathy associated with Chlamydia trachomatis infection. J Intern Med 229, 289–291

Oldstone MB (1987) Molecular mimicry and autoimmune disease [published erratum appears in Cell 1987 Dec 4;51(5):878]. Cell 50, 819–820

Ossewaarde JM, Feskens EJM, DeVries A, Vallinga CE, Kromhout D (1998) Chlamydia pneumoniae is a risk factor for coronary heart disease in symptom-free elderly men, but Helicobacter pylori and cytomegalovirus are not. Epidemiology and Infection. 120, 93–99

Penninger JM, Neu N, Bachmaier K (1996) A genetic map of autoimmune heart diseases. The Immunologist, 131–141

Penninger JM, Neu N, Timms E, Wallace VA, Koh DR, Kishihara K, Pummerer C, Mak TW (1993). Induction of experimental autoimmune myocarditis in mice lacking CD4 or CD8 molecules. J Exp Med. 178, 1837–1842

Pummerer C, Berger P, Fruhwirth M, Ofner C, Neu N (1991) Cellular infiltrate, major histocompatibility antigen expression and immunopathogenic mechanisms in cardiac myosin-induced myocarditis. Lab Invest. 65, 538–547

Pummerer CL, Grassl G, Sauer M, Bachmaier KV, Penninger JM, Neu N (1996) Cardiac myosin-induced myocarditis: Target recognition by autoreactive T cells requires prior activation of cardiac interstitial cells. Lab Invest. 74, 845–852

Pummerer CL, Luze K, Grassl G, Bachmaier K, Offner F, Burrell SK, Lenz DM, Zamborelli TJ, Penninger JM, Neu N (1996) Identification of cardiac myosin peptides capable of inducing autoimmune myocarditis in BALB/c mice. J Clin Invest. 97, 2057–2062

Ridker PM, Kundsin RB, Stampfer MJ, Poulin S, Hennekens CH (1999) Prospective study of Chlamydia pneumoniae IgG seropositivity and risks of future myocardial infarction. Circulation 99, 1161–1164

Rose NR (1996) Myocarditis: from infection to autoimmunity. The Immunologist, 67–75

Rose NR, Herskowitz A, Neumann DA, Neu N (1988) Autoimmune myocarditis: A paradigm of post-infection autoimmune disease. Immunol Today. 9, 117–120

Saikku P, Leinonen M, Mattila K, Ekman MR, Nieminen MS, Makela PH, Huttunen JK, Valtonen V (1988) Serological evidence of an association of a novel Chlamydia, TWAR, with chronic coronary heart disease and acute myocardial infarction. Lancet 2, 983–986

Smith SC, Allen PM (1992) Expression of myosin-class II major histocompatibility complexes in the normal myocardium occurs before induction of autoimmune myocarditis. Proc Nat Acad Sci USA. 89, 9131–9135

Stokes T (1997) Screening for Chlamydia in general practice: a literature review and summary of the evidence. J Public Health Med 19, 222–232

Wegmann KW, Zhao W, Griffin AC, Hickey WF (1994) Identification of myocarditogenic peptides derived from cardiac myosin capable of inducing experimental allergic myocarditis in the Lewis rat. The utility of a class II binding motif in selecting self-reactive peptides. J Immunol 153, 892–900

Woodruff JF (1980) Viral myocarditis. A review. Am J Pathol 101, 425–484

Zabriskie JB, Friedman JE (1983) The role of heart binding antibodies in rheumatic fever. Adv Exp Med Biol 161, 457–470

Printing (Computer to Film): Saladruck Berlin
Binding: Stürtz AG, Würzburg